MIND MATTERS

Setting the Stage for Satisfying Clinical Service

A Personal Essay

Ellen-Marie Silverman, Ph.D.

The anecdote shared by Jack Kornfield about listening sensitively (Kornfield, J.,2003.

The Inner Art of Meditation. Boulder, Colorado: Sounds True, Inc.) on p. 87 and

the anecdote shared by Pema Chödrön about re-imaging (Chödrön, P., 2005. *Getting Unstuck*.

Boulder, Colorado: Sounds True, Inc.) on p. 43 are used with permission from

Sounds True, Inc., www.soundstrue.com.

I have included numerous accounts of exchanges with clients, co-workers, students,

family, and friends to whom I have given fictitious names here. And I have altered certain

aspects of those exchanges to further disguise their individual identities. But this, in no way,

changed the meaning those encounters held and hold for me.

ISBN: 1-4392-2931-7
ISBN-13: 9781439229316

Library of Congress Control No. 2009901426

Visit www.booksurge.com to order additional copies

Also by Ellen-Marie Silverman

Jason's Secret

"We do not see things as they really are. We see things as we are."

- - - Anäis Nin, Diarist, Writer

TABLE OF CONTENTS

Introduction   1

    The Genesis of the Book   1

    Self-Knowledge   1

    How to Read the Book   3

    Personal Application   4

    Like Clients and Colleagues   6

    Statement of Appreciation   6

Part I Our Beliefs / Our Behaviors   9

1. Our Belief-Behavior Link: A Petite Primer   11

    Beliefs and Behaviors   11

    Projection   12

    Expectations   13

    Transference   14

    Counter-transference   15

    Clinical Examples   17

    Mike   18

    Sr. Anne   18

    Core Beliefs   20

    Transactional Analysis   24

    Uncovering Core Beliefs   26

    Asking and Answering *Why?*   26

    Example 1: The Need for Practice   27

    Example 2: Honor Intuition and Common Sense 29

    A Note About the Process   31

    Practicing Mindfulness   31

    Other Tools   34

Core Beliefs and Professed Beliefs   34

The Challenge of Desired Personal Change   37

Changing Our Beliefs to Change Our Behavior   38

Changing Our Behavior to Change Our Beliefs   39

Application to Speech-Language Pathology   39

Balance   40

Managing Desired Personal Change   41

Ongoing Self-Reflection   41

Relating with Kindness and Compassion   42

Kindness Differs from Indulgence   45

Compassion Differs from Sympathy   46

Part II Beliefs That Facilitate Desired Change   47

2. Rescuing, No. Partnering, Yes   49

The Pitfalls of Rescuing   49

Rescuing as an Unproductive Lifestyle   49

Rescuing as Distinct from Partnering   51

Rescuing As It Is   54

Invitations to Rescue   54

The Rescue Dance   60

Partnering As It Is   61

The Three P's that Increase Therapist Effectiveness   63

Potency   63

Protection   65

Permission   65

Contracting as a Structure for Partnering   67

Why Contract?   69

Why Negotiate?   69

3. We Are What We Need   71

    The Avoidable Path to Burn-Out   71

    Self-Awareness   72

    Consequences of Seeking Others' Validation of Our Worth   72

    Clinical Decision-Making   73

    Playing Politics   73

    Self-Acceptance   77

    We Are OK   78

    Self-Confidence   80

    The Elevation Effect   80

4. Understanding Trumps Knowing   83

    Six Degrees of Kevin Bacon   83

    Clients   84

    Full-Body Attending   86

    Attending Encourages Healing   86

    Hearing   87

    Seeing   88

    Our Fixation with Appearance   90

    Mind Over Matter   93

    Sensing   94

    Intuitive Communication   96

    Empathy   98

    Us-ness   99

    What Is   101

    Guard-All   102

    Compassion   105

    Me First   105

5. Right and Wrong I: What Is   107

    Pentimento   110

    What's Right   111

    More Than We Customarily Acknowledge   111

    Expressions of Gratitude   111

    What's Wrong   112

    We're Not the Only Ones   112

    An Invitation to Learn   113

    What About Therapy?   115

    Balance   116

    Starting With Ourselves   117

    Drawing on Strengths to Fashion New Skills   119

    Beliefs As Architects   122

6. Right and Wrong II: Harmonizing   125

    I'm Right; You're Wrong. Lose-Lose   125

    Effect on Professional Practice   126

    Point of View   128

    What Does Anger Have to Do With It?   131

    Causes and Solutions   133

    Coming Together   135

    Filial Imprinting   138

    A "By the Way"   140

Part III Establishing Change   143

7. Slowing Down to Strengthen Endurance   145

    Patience and Skill-Building   145

    The Fruits of Patience   148

    We Always Have a Choice   150

    Ways of Slowing Down   150

Meditation 152

The Genesis and Brief History of a Practice 152

Developing a Work-Related Personal Practice 154

Sitting and Moving 155

Personal Journaling 156

Asking and Answering "Why?" 157

Journaling Gratitude 158

Drawing and Painting 159

Realism 160

Drawing From Two Different Mind-Sets 160

Coda 163

Appendix A: 165

Creating Conditions for Change 167

Appendix B: 175

Learning to Sit 177

Appendix C: 181

Happily Ever After 183

End Notes 189

References 193

About The Author 203

Index 205

INTRODUCTION

THE GENESIS OF THE BOOK

What do you do after you have practiced speech-language pathology for more than 40 years because you have a passion to help people communicate? I asked myself that question recently, and answered: *Write a book. Share what you learned.*

Knowing I was one of few (e.g., Hinckley, 2007; Silverman, 2008b; 2006b; 2003a; 2001b; 2000) speech-language pathologists addressing clinicians' self-knowledge as a major clinical variable, I believed writing about the importance of ongoing self-reflection worthy of at least a few more years of work. Distilled, the message would be: *Our personal core beliefs drive our professional practice and help determine whether or not we develop satisfying and long-lived careers (e.g., Silverman, 2008b).* These primal beliefs, residing just below conscious awareness, fashion our relationships, which are our most potent clinical tool (e.g., Moore, 2006; Silverman, 2006b). Detecting and examining them helps us create relationships with clients and caregivers, as well as with colleagues and students, that support growth, theirs and ours (e.g., Richo, 2008). This insight reflects the most valuable insight I learned from working as a therapist.

But don't worry. *Mind Matters* isn't a painfully personal rant or romp about coming of age as a clinician, although I do include anecdotes from my career and life. It is an account of why and how to excavate and analyze personal core beliefs and of the adoption and cultivation of certain selected, organizing beliefs to sharpen clinical practice. With references to more than 145 books, periodicals, audio CD's, videos, and DVD's, many of which describe applicable concepts and tools, it becomes apparent that what I learned others have as well. Altogether, an ancillary thesis is: Incorporating beliefs and practices, already successfully applied by physicians, psychologists, social workers, and clergy to enliven, hone, and make more relevant their service, also increases the effectiveness of our own while revealing the similarity of our complementary practices and concerns.

SELF-KNOWEDGE

That our beliefs affect our thoughts and emotions and fashion our behavior is hardly a novel thought. But appreciating the porous connection between personal beliefs and professional conduct was a revelatory insight for me. I, as others I have known, have been encouraged to believe we can draw a solid line of demarcation between our personal beliefs and our professional conduct, yet I have observed this belief to be faulty. While we may think we can provide equal treatment for all, as stipulated by our profession's Code of Ethics, we can not when, for example, we personally believe people practicing a particular religion or from a certain culture, race, or ethnic group or with a particular gender identification or sexual orientation are incapable of fully appreciating or deserving of what we have to offer. When we covertly despise and, thereby, diminish another, we withhold to some degree and manner the knowledge, skill, and compassion we would, otherwise, apply to help them meet their communication, cognitive, literacy, and swallowing needs. Training has alerted most of us to the detrimental effects arising from holding bigoted views. But few of us recognize the magnitude of disarray that can arise from acting on the seemingly less odious and more pervasive beliefs we tacitly seem to champion as appropriate to the novice therapist's role. For instance, *when we encourage each other to believe, that during clinical decision-making with legally competent clients and caregivers, we alone know what is best for them, we are placing our need to be right before their need to be helped (e.g., Silverman, 2003c)* . Acting as though we, more than clients and caregivers, know what they want and need and in what sequence may help us feel strong as *newbies* when we, otherwise, may feel uncertain and vulnerable, but that belief rarely leads us to the payoff they or we desire (e.g., Sohan, 2008). Dominating people in the guise of helping them usually encourages them to feel powerless and, ultimately, to rebel. When we metaphorically move clients and caregivers through treatment regimes as though they were sacks of potatoes to be carted from farm field to market to kitchen table, they often refuse to perform tasks, skip sessions, avoid meetings, and, ultimately, quit in an untimely and unpleasant manner because we offended them by discounting their desire and ability to take responsibility for meeting their needs with our help. If so, they may delay or resist seeking further professional help. That could crystallize their problem-related beliefs and behaviors, making eventual attempts to change them more challenging and less successful than they, otherwise, might have been.

And we can be hurt as well by acting on the belief that, in matters of clinical decision-making, we know best. As we watch clients and caregivers quietly or loudly storm out of treatment relationships they believe failed them primarily because they did not feel validated by us, we, in turn, feel rejected, hurt, and angered because we believe we were misunderstood by them. We know we did our best. So, to have our best thrown back at us as worthless or, even, hurtful and harmful prompts us to take action to assuage our hurt. For many of us, that involves hardening our hearts to remaining and future clients and caregivers. By choosing to feel less, we momentarily hurt less, but we pay a high price for that short-lived relief. We become less empathetic and increasingly remote and mechanical. As we dissociate from our unpleasant feelings, we increase our vulnerability to professional burn-out, decreasing our possibility for enjoying the long-lived, satisfying career for which we had enthusiastically and painstakingly prepared. Such is the potentially destructive fall-out for us all when we choose to believe we know more than clients and caregivers about their needs and how to meet them.

If, instead, we harbor the belief that our truth is simply our point-of-view and no more or no less important than the truth of clients, caregivers, colleagues, students, supervisors, and employers with whom we interact, we can freely collaborate to address the concerns and challenges we collectively face without incurring the risks of client rebellion or professional burn-out. *Recognizing that what we personally believe about ourselves, others, and the world around us is as important to our clinical service as our clinical skill and knowledge elevates our personal and professional effectiveness.* We function, after all, as entire human beings. What we personally believe influences whatever we do and say wherever we are and with whomever we are with, as sensitivity training regarding our attitude and response toward individuals of an identified gender, race, culture, class, and/or physical, mental, or emotional challenge abundantly demonstrates.

HOW TO READ THE BOOK

Mind Matters consists of seven chapters, five of which, i.e., Chapters 2 through 6 respectively, "Partnering Yes; Rescuing, No," "What Are What We Need," "Understanding Trumps Knowing," "Right & Wrong I: What Is," and "Right & Wrong II: Harmonizing," amplify the central point introduced in Chapter 1, "Our Belief-Behavior Link: A Petite Primer," namely, that *personal beliefs matter in professional practice.* The final chapter, Chapter 7, "Slowing Down To Strengthen Endurance" highlights the role of patience in the management of change. Patience helps us to be kinder to ourselves and others to create a climate that fosters growth. Without it, insight suffers and desired change can irredeemably veer off-course.

This book concludes with three appendixes. Appendix A and Appendix C each contain a paper I presented at the International Stuttering Awareness Day Online Conference chaired by Prof. Judith Kuster at Minnesota State University, Mankato. Appendix A, "Creating Conditions for Change," presented in 2007, addresses fundamental aspects of change important for clinicians to consider when addressing clients' and caregivers' needs, particularly those with stuttering problems. Appendix C, "Happily Ever After," presented in 2008, considers the desire for long-lasting happiness to be the primary motivation for clients and caregivers seeking therapy to resolve communication and swallow problems and outlines how we can best help them in that quest. Appendix B, "Learning to Sit," presents, in narrative form, the fluid nature of my developing meditation practice, including antecedents and consequences, to highlight the personal, even idiosyncratic nature of the process, within which I have participated off-and-on for almost 30 years, that requires expenditure of effort and a generous application of patience and persistence.

Taking time to identify our *core beliefs*, which we first established as children and which continue to function into adulthood as the source of many of our thoughts and actions, permits us to assess their current appropriateness to both our professional development and continuing personal growth. Suggestions for ways to identify, examine, and analyze them appear in Chapters 1 and 7 which also provide specific direction for achieving the calm, penetrating mind-state essential to self-assessment through the practice of mindfulness. When we thoroughly consider the legitimacy of a core belief, we can decide whether to maintain, modify, or abandon it. Chapters 2 through 6 individually highlight particular beliefs derived from my experience as a clinician and as a transactional analysis trainee that

I have found critical to my professional development. Perhaps, some are familiar and some are not. At any rate, cultivating some or all of them, i.e., the value of partnering clients, the reality of self-sufficiency, the relevance and power of compassionate understanding, and the relativity of "right" and "wrong" (addressed across two adjacent chapters, 5 and 6), can enhance clinical effectiveness and work satisfaction as well as the planning, conduct, and assessment of research studies. Each chapter from Chapter 2 through Chapter 6 offers guidance for incorporating and expressing these beliefs in clinical work. Their application to research can be inferred from their contribution to clinical practice since the nature of an ethical clinical relationship between clinician and client resembles an ethical research relationship between experimenter and subject.

As far as where to start reading *Mind Matters* and in what order to continue, I see no reason why that cannot reflect individual choice. But, I should mention, I did sequence the chapters to establish a momentum to quietly stimulate and gently shepherd personal professional change to reach a crescendo in the "Right and Wrong" chapters, i.e., 5 and 6. Of course, if you have purchased this volume for a class, seminar, or individual study upon the direction of an instructor or mentor who knows you better than I and who has made a personal decision about the order in which to introduce you to the content for your personal benefit, then the matter is settled.

PERSONAL APPLICATION

As I reflect upon the nature of *Mind Matters*, I recognize the book fits the category of a style manual more so than, say, a fashion statement. Style endures. Fashions come and go. We eventually learn this as we shop for clothes, shoes, and accessories, arrange our hair, and decorate our abodes. While it may seem quicker and even more exciting to purchase the current fad and adopt the latest craze than come to know ourselves well enough to seek out the style which communicates our essence, eventually this emotionally-driven, occasionally frenzied, activity to conform to some media-defined ideal becomes tiresome. It fails to satisfy our innate desire to be who we are. So, we learn to settle down, to identify and develop our attractive features and express them in our attire and surroundings. In short, we develop style.

Similarly, we come to recognize that keeping up-to-date in our professional reading and taking the most current seminars and workshops to become acquainted with fashionable testing and treatment procedures may only teach us to perform new tasks rather than serve as increasingly well-rounded clinicians. To do that, we need to shine as the individuals we are, which we do, in part, by adopting the ongoing practice of identifying, examining, and analyzing our core beliefs and by cultivating helpful new ones. This essential professional practice helps us exhibit a stable, energetic presence that encourages desirable growth, ours and that of those around us. It is presence, after all, which, more than anything we can say or do, facilitates desirable change (e.g., Soygal, 2005; Kornfield, 2003; Silverman, 2006b) enabling us to increasingly relate to one another as more of a help than a nuisance (Wiegela, 1996) to become the clinician we wish to be.

If you wonder how you may put this book to best use for yourself, since, unlike many books for clinicians, *Mind Matters is written for you to apply to your own personal and related professional growth process*, then my suggestions, presented in Chapter 7, are to: 1) Develop a personal mindfulness practice. 2) Keep a daily or, at least, a weekly, journal to reflect on a particularly pleasant or unpleasant experience as a basis for identifying core beliefs impacting on you and your work by applying the method illustrated in Chapter 1 and another one identifying perceived strengths. And 3) Create at least one realistic drawing or painting every month.

Mindfulness Practice

While many forms of mindfulness practice exist, mindfulness meditation or *vipassana* practice, (e.g., Kabat-Zinn, 2005; 1995) helps us to become increasingly acquainted with the working of our mind. This knowledge helps us monitor in real-time our almost continuous self-talk associated with our core beliefs. By doing that, we become increasingly skilled at identifying unhelpful messages we send ourselves before they compel us to act and feel in habitual ways we wish to discontinue as well as detecting helpful messages we wish to act upon in a timely manner to increase our effectiveness and satisfaction.

Personal Journaling

Explicit journaling helps make core beliefs, which reside just below the surface of our ordinary waking consciousness, more recognizable than analysis and contemplation alone. When we put our perceptions into words we can see and consider, we are likely to be more accurate and thorough in our self-reflection and to take appropriate, corrective action as needed. Chapter 1 illustrates a deceptively simple, yet unfailingly effective, approach to journaling as a basis for excavating core beliefs. It involves our repetitive asking and answering, *"Why?"* This method is re-visited in Chapter 7, which also includes an approach to journaling that identifies perceived personal strengths. Combined, the two practices help balance our self-view.

Drawing and Painting

By developing the attitude and manner of attention required to draw and paint realistically, we learn to relate more directly to that which is outside ourselves free of the concepts and labels we subconsciously and customarily apply to what we perceive. For instance, instead of drawing the ash tree before us as a vertical rectangle perpendicular to the ground with an orb of green atop as we might if we applied the concept "This is how to draw a tree." we learned in first grade, we notice and represent the curvature of the trunk, the projection of the branches, and the color, density, and robustness of the foliage as the tree actually presents itself. By so doing, we relate to our subject, the ash tree, in an unmediated or, direct, way devoid of the blinders concepts place on experience. As we relate ever more directly to our subject, our rendering of it becomes increasingly truer. And our wisdom grows. Learning to relate to what actually is situated before us rather than an *a priori* notion of what we think is there slowly transfers into our approach to life in general, including our clinical and research relationships.

LIKE CLIENTS AND COLLEAGUES

As a young speech-language pathologist, I believed my work differed from that of practioners in other helping professions. But, as I worked as a member of teams committed to meeting the needs of autistic children, traumatically brain-injured young adults, and geriatric patients, I recognized the similarity of the work many of us do. Like teachers, psychologists, physical therapists, occupational therapists, social workers, physicians, nurses, and others, speech-language pathologists accept responsibility for effectively managing client change. We each identify what clients and caregivers might change, the tools they need to do that, and the motivational requirements necessary to achieve those goals.

And, just as the basic nature of the job we as speech-language pathologists perform corresponds to the essential nature of the job carried-out by colleagues in other professions, so, too, does our monitoring and modifying of our manner of interacting with our self and others mirror the basic activity clients and caregivers. We, like they, recognize, accept, and analyze how we are and choose to think and act as we wish to be, applying patience and endurance to the establishment of new ways of thinking and behaving. With that in mind, I hope the content of *Mind Matters* serves as a reminder to recall and appreciate the fact we all are more alike than different in our deeply held aspirations to be happy and free of suffering. Recognizing that helps us elevate the level of compassion we infuse into our life and work.

STATEMENT OF APPRECIATION

I owe a tremendous debt to all the teachers, students, clients, caregivers, colleagues, family, friends, employers, and employees alike with whom I have been privileged to share pleasant experiences and those with whom I have experienced discord, which was, in fact, a most demanding and elegant teacher. All helped me broaden and steady my vision and act more compassionately, and it is to all of them that I dedicate this book. Those who I have taught formally and informally, including my daughter Catherine Bette Silverman Thomas, have brought much insight into my life, and, to them, too, I dedicate this book. May what I have written about what I have learned help you help others. If so, please pay it forward.

I have included numerous accounts of exchanges with clients, co-workers, students, family, and friends to whom I have given fictitious names here. And I have altered certain aspects of those exchanges to further disguise their individual identities. But this, in no way, changed the meaning those encounters held and hold for me. The bulk of clinical anecdotes included come from my experience with adults experiencing cognitive, memory, language, stuttering, and voice problems.

This book is loosely based on a paper I presented at the 9th Annual International Stuttering Awareness Day (ISAD) Online Conference in October in 2006, entitled, *Mind Matters* (Silverman, 2006c). The Conference, chaired by Prof. Judith Kuster, Minnesota State University, Mankato, has been archived and is freely available at www.mnsu.edu/comdis/kuster/stutter.html where the paper, posts made to it, and my responses to the posts all can be read.

PART I

OUR BELIEFS / OUR BEHAVIORS

This section affords a glimpse into the belief-behavior connection that influences our work as clinicians, researchers, and teachers. As professionals, we act based upon what we believe to be true about ourselves, others, and the world around us as much as upon what we believe are sound professional opinions concerning cause and intervention. Serving well depends upon examining our personal core beliefs as we do our professional opinions. Since our core beliefs elude casual detection, identifying them involves dedicated, ongoing self-reflection. The process of probing why we acted as we did following encounters that leave us feeling baffled, saddened, or pleased brings these critical beliefs into conscious awareness. The simple, direct, and powerful tool for excavating them introduced here encores in Chapter 7.

1   OUR BELIEF-BEHAVIOR LINK: A PETITE PRIMER

"As a man thinketh in his heart, so is he. "

- - - *Proverbs 23:7*

Some time ago, I came to the realization that the way we conduct ourselves as therapists[1] is as much an outgrowth of our beliefs about ourselves, others, and society as it is a function of the specific theoretical orientations and diagnostic and therapeutic skills we acquire and, possibly, more so. To say this somewhat differently: I believe what we believe is more important than anything we may do. And I think our clients[2] think so, too. Research findings support this presumption. Observations of groups of student and practicing therapists (e.g., Moore, 2006; Silverman, 2003a; Crane, et al., 1986) have documented that the more empathetic the therapist appears to the client, the more successful the therapy experience for the client. In fact, Moore (2006) noted that, in her experience, those clients with whom she believed she had been empathetic reported satisfaction with their treatment experience with her even when they had not reached their treatment goals.   This observation is consistent with Daniel Goleman's (2006a) belief that empathy is hard-wired into our brains. It is, in fact, unnatural for us to view others as "its" to be manipulated and controlled, as has been encouraged by the misapplication of empirical science methodologies to clinical concerns (Silverman, 2001). Given that our behavior stems from our beliefs, adopting an ongoing practice of identifying our core beliefs and cultivating helpful ones become an essential, evolving task for both students and practicing professionals. That is what this book is about.

BELIEFS AND BEHAVIORS

We all relate differently to calm, thoughtful, attentive professionals intent on listening to us than we do to those who appear annoyed, distracted, and distant. We and our clients also are more likely to disclose our concerns, needs, hopes, and fears to therapists who listen to us without judgment and project kindness and than we are to those who repeatedly interrupt and criticize us. And we are no more likely to place our trust and open our hearts and minds to therapists who appear uncomfortable than we are to those who seem hostile. More than our feelings about our meetings with therapists are affected by their behavior. Our behavior is, too. How we perceive and interact with those who serve us ultimately determines whether or not we view the total experience as positive (e.g., Charon, 2006; Silverman, 2006b; 2000).

As therapists, we tend to feel satisfied, even elated, when our clients and their caregivers report satisfaction with our efforts on their behalf. That is the very feeling, or payoff, we desire and, for most of us, the experience for which we prepared so hard for so long to experience. Yet as hard as we work, as much as we learn, we do not always experience this feeling. Sometimes we feel hurt and dismay when clients resist our probing for critical background information, or fail to respond enthusiastically or at all to our treatment strategies and recommendations, or quit, especially when they do so abruptly and harshly, such as by flaming email, as was the recent experience of one therapist I know. We may respond to such disappointments by developing self-protective, pull-back stances to emotionally distance ourselves from future clients and the sense of failure working with them may bring. We may blame our clients for our lack of perceived success. We may tell ourselves and our clients they did not try hard enough; that they were impatient and gave up too soon; that they lacked motivation; and so forth, without carefully assessing the contribution of our own motivation and conduct to the painful outcome because we were unaware of the need to engage in the process and unfamiliar with the tools involved. Not to practice ongoing self-reflection deprives us of the opportunity to grow, which can lead to cynicism and ignite professional burn-out, leaving bitterness, resentment, and confusion in our wake.

Reacting to our clients' seeming dissatisfaction with our work by emotionally distancing ourselves from them is, unfortunately, a common response that does more harm than good. Withholding our kindness, empathy, and compassion to protect ourselves from possible emotional hurt only increases the possibility of further rejection and failure. Instead, we can help both ourselves and our present and future clients by carefully considering what may be motivating our clients to act toward us in such unwelcome ways and respond constructively to that understanding. Perhaps, they relate to us that way because of experiences they have had in life in general based on their gender, family, cultural, societal, and generational happenstance that do not seem to resonate for them within our medical or educational practice. Perhaps, they relate that way because of their experience with other helping professionals who left them feeling hopeless, even worthless. And, perhaps, they relate that way if we came across as more concerned with administering tests and surveys and charting target behaviors than relating to them as individuals (Moore, 2006; Silverman, 2003a).

Projection

"We do not see things as they really are. We see things as we are."

- - - *Anaïs Nin, Writer, Diarist*

We do not unilaterally determine how clients perceive us. We may do all we can to cultivate beliefs that promote growth to gain client and caregiver confidence and trust, but that does not mean they will receive our efforts as we intended them. Nor may we always see our clients as the individuals they truly are. Unless and until we recognize these possibilities and become acquainted with our core beliefs, will we not be able to relate to others as they genuinely are. Instead, we will relate to them as projections of our own unresolved needs, to which they will respond as their own projections guide them.

Unrecognized *expectations* and transference of emotions from earlier experiences and relationships to the present one through the unconscious dynamics of *transference* and *counter-transference* coax us and our clients into relating to each other as phantoms rather than the people we actually are (e.g., Richo, 2008).

Expectations

> *". . . I am not in this world to live up to your expectations,*
>
> *and you are not in this world to live up to mine. . . "*
>
> - - - *Fritz Perls*, Founder, *GestaltTherapy*

Clients, at times, reject our best efforts because of their life experience, what they perceive ours to be, and the beliefs they hold about how to be with us. Clients almost always have certain expectations about how it will be for them working with us as professionals and individuals, and we will have certain expectations about how it may be for us to be working with them as clients and as individuals. For instance, adults who have had stuttering problems since they were children and may have experienced only disappointing outcomes since they first experienced speech therapy as children, may expect once again to experience a sense of personal failure by working with yet another speech therapist. Even though they seek treatment, they may be quite unwilling to commit fully to the process. Some may be distrustful and uncomfortable relating to individuals of a certain race, culture, gender, age, and/or socio-economic status which we represent and expect disrespect even incompetence from us until they are willing to challenge the *stereotype* they hold for groups we represent. Some may be disheartened by experiences with the educational or healthcare systems in which they encounter us, and, initially, at least, unwilling to expect that any professional employee in the system really wants to help them. Of course, it is equally possible that clients may have unreasonably high expectations of what we can do for them if we use the title "Dr," if we work at a prestigious medical faculty or within a university clinic, or if they were recommended to us by someone who had been exceptionally satisfied with our work.

We may tend to harbor expectations about clients with life experience different from our own. We may expect individuals from social-cultural-economic-generational backgrounds other than our own to not know what we know, to know more than we know, or to value or not value what we do, encouraging us to consider our knowledge, experience, and values superior or inferior to theirs. We may expect clients with a particular diagnosis, say traumatic brain injury, to have similar, if not the same, reasons for participating in outpatient rehabilitation and fail to take fully into account their individual goals and desires. Or, for instance, we may expect to fail working with clients with certain diagnoses and rationalize refusing them treatment. It is not uncommon, for example, for speech therapists, who, as students and then as professionals, may have had little to no experience working with children who have stuttering problems to be apprehensive about working with them and their caregivers. We may harbor limited expectations for individuals who have not graduated from high school, have a history of substance abuse, are HIV positive, and so forth. *We are human beings first and foremost, so we can expect ourselves to hold certain limiting expectations about the clients we work with as we do for ourselves.* Once we acknowledge that, we can begin the process of identifying and releasing beliefs that spawn such expectations.

Transference

We need to deeply consider that it is not unusual for clients to subconsciously relate to us as though we were an adult with whom they related as a child (e.g., Richo, 2008). By transferring their as yet unresolved emotional reactions to that individual, usually a parent, to us, they engage in what has been called transference (e.g., Maroda, 1991). For example, if we are female, that happenstance alone may be sufficient for a client to relate to us as though we were their mother, warm, friendly, and endlessly forgiving, or, possibly, distant, aloof, and forever critical. More than once, for example, preschool and school-age clients have called me "Mommy" while involved in an activity we were sharing. When they heard themselves say that, all reacted by shaking their heads as if saying, "No, no. That's not right!" laughing, or countering with some embarrassment, "I mean, Ellen." But all, nevertheless, at the subconscious level, considered me "Mommy" at the time or they would not have referred to me as such. With older clients, transference behaviors rarely are that obvious. As we carefully examine our beliefs, thoughts, motives, feelings, and behaviors working with a client and discern they do not of themselves warrant the hostile or obsequious responses a client is making toward us, we probably can conclude they are transferring unresolved feelings from an earlier relationship to us. If such behavior does not seem to be interfering with the client's progress, we can merely note it for what it is, if it is tolerable, and continue the current treatment program. But if the transference behaviors appear to be deflecting the client from achieving otherwise achievable goals, we need to consider helping the client learn to relate to us as the person we are and not as, for example, their *ersatz* mother or ex-partner (Maroda, 1991).

When I was working as a senior therapist and team leader in an outpatient rehabilitation program for young adults with traumatic brain injury, I had a clinical relationship tainted by transference issues I needed to address. That relationship was with a male I'll call Charles. Charles was the leader of a local rock band with a fast-growing following. In his early 30's with a reputation as a dedicated womanizer, he allegedly became brain-injured as the result of being beaten unconscious by an unknown assailant wielding a baseball bat seeking revenge for Charles' seduction of his wife. When I first met Charles, I immediately thought how little-boy cute he was, a thought I probably silently broadcast since I do not have a poker-face. That may have encouraged him to behave flirtatiously toward me, which he apparently did with all women who were alive and had teeth. I did not respond to his seductive facial expressions and body language except, perhaps, by showing signs of annoyance while covertly appreciating receiving romantic-like attention from such a cute younger guy. My conflicted feelings may have been quite apparent to him and may be the reason he continued relating to me in this professionally unwelcome manner. After several sessions, I told him directly and simply that flirting with the therapist was unacceptable. He nodded in agreement, and, from then on he concentrated on achieving his speech, language, and cognitive goals, and was dismissed after successfully accomplishing them all. I do not know whether his response to what I said led to situational repression of his flirtatious behavior or reflected a genuine understanding of the fact that it is possible and appropriate to relate to a woman under certain circumstances without viewing her as a potential score. But, at a pragmatic level, within the context of our relationship, my redirection of his seemingly automatically choreographed emotional response to me was effective. He left a better communicator, and I was able to direct all my attention when I worked with him to his speech, communicative, and cognitive needs.

Transference differs from *stereotyping*. When we respond to another in a stereotypical way, we relate to them as a member of group we find acceptable, or not. When we exhibit transference, we are relating to the person with us as an individual, just not as the individual they actually are. Instead, we use the current relationship to symbolically relate to someone from our past for whom we have had strong feelings that remain unresolved. So, metaphorically speaking, when we engage in the process of transference, we place a mask resembling the other person over the face of the person with whom we currently are in relationship to relive the emotional nature of the earlier relationship and, perhaps, resolve it.

Transference is a common feature of all interpersonal relationships, including teaching and supervising, mentoring, managing employees, parenting, partnering, and friendships. Skillfully managing transference can be challenging unless we see it for what it is and redirect the transference behaviors in a timely manner with warmth and kindness to the others involved and to ourselves. Applying humor softens the process and can make it more agreeable.

Counter-transference

Sometimes we relate to our clients not as who they are but as people we have known. Like transference this common, subconscious response arises when the traits and attributes of a client remind us of an individual with whom we have not yet reconciled a powerful, emotional connection. So, instead of relating to a particular client as the individual himself or herself, we relate to that client as if he or she was an older deceased brother, a former boyfriend, a childhood friend, the schoolyard bully, our mother, and so forth. When classroom teachers participate in sexual relationships with current students, they may not be relating to the student but to a phantom lover, a particularly sad misperception. Subconsciously relating to a client as someone the client resembles rather than the client himself or herself is called *counter-transference* (e.g., Maroda, 1991), and , like transference, counter-transference commonly occurs in all relationships including helping ones and is a possibility we need to prepare to detect and skillfully manage.

I experienced counter-transference for the first time as a speech therapist when I was 21 years old, although I did not consciously realize that until several years later. The experience occurred in 1964, when I began my first position as a staff speech correctionist, the earlier designation for speech pathologists, with a demonstration project for preschool autistic children and their parents. Like other professionals, we, too, considered autism a psychiatric disorder caused by emotionally distant parents, especially educated mothers, who communicated poorly with their children causing them to feel rejected. Prior to assuming the position, I had almost no professional experience working with parents of young children and, as most speech therapists at the time, almost no formal instruction about the art and science of constructing helping relationships.

From the first day on the job, I detested the mothers of my clients for what I self-righteously assumed they had done to their children. And I felt pleasure doing so! I had no compassion for any of these, what I now know, frightened, anxious women. I avoided or cut short conversations with them, partly because, being new, I was not sure what to say and primarily because I despised these women for harming their own children. I worked quite well with the children themselves. Neither my supervisor nor any other staff member criticized my paltry, cruel interactions with their mothers.

Years later, well into my career, I realized I had not been relating to my clients' mothers as the individuals they were: I was relating to them as if they were my own mother and stepmother. My mother died at home from a stroke late one evening as I watched the process unfold. I was three years old. My next memory was of my father, unskilled in dealing with feelings, telling me the next day why she was gone. He joined me in the bathroom as I sat on the toilet urinating Balanced on the rim of the tub across from where I sat, hunched over and smoking a cigarette, and looking at the cold, tiled floor, he muttered that my mother had gone to Heaven. Then he quickly walked away leaving a mist of white-grey tobacco smoke before me. He had not hugged me. He had not kissed me. He had not even looked me in the eye. He said what he had to say and left. I did not know what Heaven was. All I knew was that my mother was gone, and I felt horribly, painfully alone in the world and terrified because of that. As a three-year-old and for many years thereafter, I thought my mother would return if I was good enough. Of course, she never did, and I both missed and hated her for leaving. A year later, my father brought me back home from an aunt and uncle's house where he had placed me that day. A woman I did not know was there, and he told me she was my new mother. From that day on, she regularly and fiercely abused me, physically, mentally, and emotionally.

When I began working on the autism project, the unrecognized, unprocessed grief and rage I felt toward my mother and stepmother surfaced with the mothers who had supposedly emotionally abandoned their children. I subconsciously turned them into my mother and stepmother to deal with my own still raw pain, 18 years after my mother died. Sadly, by shunning the mothers as I had, I undoubtedly caused additional and unnecessary suffering for at least some and, as a consequence, their children as well, instead of soothing their pain, as I, who had been hired as a healer, was expected to do. I can not reverse whatever hurt I caused these already hurting women and their children, but I now carefully reflect on the basis for all strong feelings I have for my clients and their caregivers and act accordingly. And I forgive myself when I discover I have attended to my needs more than theirs.

Relationship is our most important clinical tool (Silverman, 2006b). When a client seems to misunderstand us, and treatment is going badly or when we feel strongly toward a client in some manner, and treatment is suffering, we need to calmly reconsider our verbal and non-verbal behavior and examine our intent. If we consider the client's or caregiver's manner of relating to us to be inappropriate, and we are not succeeding in our efforts to redirect the unhelpful behavior, we need to refer the client to another therapist who may be better able to establish an effective therapy relationship. Similarly, if we believe our behavior and intent toward a client is inappropriate, and we do not believe we can relate any differently at the time, we need to refer that client to another therapist more likely to relate directly and reasonably to the client. We also need to do what is necessary to suitably resolve our own needs. Recognizing the need to do so and appropriately addressing it are evidence of our increasing personal and professional maturity, even wisdom, as we grow into our fullness of being and skill and reason for praise.

Very few of us see ourselves and others as the individuals we truly are. The better acquainted we become with our interior and exterior selves, i.e. our beliefs and behaviors, the better we will come to know others and relate skillfully to them as the individuals they actually are on the inside as well as on the outside.

Clinical Examples.

Two encounters I have had with adult clients, a police officer who experienced traumatic brain injury following a collision with another motor vehicle while driving his squad car during a high speed motor vehicle chase and an elderly Roman Catholic nun who suffered brain injury after falling and hitting her head in a convent stairwell, highlight how learning to see clients as they are rather than how we think they are, or how we wish them to be, affects our usefulness to them (Silverman, 2006a; 2003a; 2000). I have summarized these experiences below beginning with a key aspect of the rehabilitation services experience of the police officer.

Mike. As a senior therapist and team leader in an outpatient rehabilitation program for young adults with traumatic brain injury, I was assigned to work with a client I'll call Mike. Mike had been the client of another speech therapist on our team the previous week or two, and, because my office/treatment suite shared a paper thin wall with hers, I could hear their daily, increasingly hostile, arguments, which I would have been able to hear even if my office had been at the opposite end of the hall. He wanted a rationale for each task she asked him to perform. She, a physically diminutive but an emotionally aggressive woman, enjoyed dominating patients, males in particular, and told him essentially that he was to do what she expected, no questions asked. He, a strapping six-foot, 200- plus pound alpha-male police sergeant, not unexpectedly, resisted her efforts to intimidate him. He asked the program manager to transfer him to another therapist. He did, and that other therapist became me.

At our first meeting, I asked him why he wanted to work with a different speech therapist, not because I did not know but because I wanted to hear his explanation. He practically exploded. His face turned red. He leaned forward until his face was inches from mine and fiercely pointed his right index finger in my direction. *"She just treated me like a piece of meet,"* he shouted. *"She just said, 'Do this. Do that.' She never once treated me like a person. Not once."* Since my style was to include all clients in decision-making, to the extent they were interested and able, working with him as an individual and partner in his rehabilitation process was not a problem for me. I explained this to him and alerted the occupational and physical therapists on our team that Mike expected to be a fully functioning team member. We worked with him that way, and he responded with enthusiasm and determination that led to considerable effort. Within six months, he was able to return to his precinct in a limited duty capacity. Several years later, I learned he had resumed patrol duty.

Sr. Anne. My experience with the aged Roman Catholic nun I'll call Sr. Anne presented somewhat differently, but it, too, reveals the problems we can create for our clients and ourselves when we see clients as we think they are rather than as they are. I worked with Sr. Anne only once, as an on-call therapist at a rehabilitation hospital when I substituted for her ailing therapist. This therapist had diagnosed Sr. Anne as *globally aphasic*, neither able to understand written or spoken language or arithmetic which prevented her from speaking, writing, or solving simple arithmetic problems. The therapist's daily treatment notes for the therapy-to-date showed no progress during naming tasks, the only skill addressed. Nursing home placement was considered as the only possibility for her.

The goal of occupational therapy was to help Sr. Anne recover basic self-care functions, such as washing herself and brushing her teeth, which the right-sided weakness caused by her brain injury had disrupted.

I met Sr. Anne and the occupational therapist for a co-therapy session that morning in the tiny bathroom of Sr. Anne's room. They had already begun. Sr. Anne, a frail, shrunken, woman, of a seemingly mild and reticent nature, sat listing to her left in a wheelchair with her upper torso bare and exposed. She held a dampened wash cloth in her left hand. She instantly evidenced awareness of my arrival by turning her head in my direction. Looking deeply into my eyes as few have, she seemed to be assessing me deeply. At first, I felt some anxiety wondering whether she would find me acceptable since her facial expression was stark. But I quickly abandoned that thought as my being filled with the tremendous pity I felt for her, so exposed, so vulnerable in the presence of two relative strangers., with at least one of which, me, uncertain how to best help her.

Then I noticed the thick lens of her glasses heavily smudged with fingerprints. I removed the frames after obtaining what I was certain was tacit approval from Sr. Anne. As I cleaned the lenses, my sense of pity escalated as I considered the irony of having to wear glasses that impaired vision. As I placed them back on her head, my brief angry reverie was interrupted by the sound of Sr. Anne's voice. She spoke directly to me, clearly and firmly, *"What I need is empathy not sympathy."* This intelligible, grammatical, and perfectly appropriate, high level statement uttered to me in a cautionary tone was not something an individual with global aphasia could do. It woke me up in more ways than one!

A short while later, as I was walking through the clients' common area in the rehabilitation unit, I noticed Sr. Anne sitting alone at a dining table staring longingly at a small styrofoam cup directly in front of her but beyond the reach of her hands now bound in gauze to prevent self-mutilation. I asked her whether she wanted to drink the juice that seemed to have been placed there for her. After a brief period of silence, she responded as distinctly and firmly as in her room, *"Yes."* she replied. Sr. Anne clearly was not globally aphasic. Her response time was somewhat slower than most. Her vision had been impaired by the dirty lenses of her glasses and may have been so for an indeterminate time. Either or both factors may have contributed to her poor scores on various speech therapy tests and tasks.

Prior to leaving the hospital, I documented these observations in the daily treatment notes section of her medical chart and in the speech therapy folder in the speech therapist's office. The Director of Rehabilitation at the hospital never again called me to work.

How could Sr. Anne have been so incorrectly diagnosed? As I observed therapists scurrying about the rehabilitation hospital that morning, it was clear to me that they behaved as though they thought their real work was to see clients to complete necessary paperwork. They saw clients, but they did not really *see* them. They related primarily to their expectations of how a client should respond to a specific task, rather than to each client as an individual. Their behavior reminded me of an Hasidic tale (Gafni, 2004), which I have modified:

A tourist noticed three men working on an urban lot where she was told a synagogue was being erected. Approaching one, she asked, What are you doing? I am a stone mason, the man answered. I cut stone. That is what I do. Turning to the second, she asked, What are you doing? I am a brick layer, the worker replied. I lay bricks. That is what I do. Addressing the remaining worker, sweeping the area with a broom, she asked, What are you doing? I am building a beautiful temple for God and the people, he answered smiling.

Many of the hospital rehabilitation staff, like the stone mason and brick layer and unlike the simple street sweeper, did not seem to appreciate the larger picture of which their work was part. They seemingly suppressed their natural instincts to touch others' lives with kind attention (Goleman, 2006) and, instead, concentrated on fulfilling the persistent, persuasive demands of the healthcare system which employed them, and that was to concentrate on generating revenue while protecting themselves and their employer from potential, costly malpractice litigation. By and large, their interactions with patients seemed incidental and mindless (e.g., Langer, 1989).

CORE BELIEFS

Core beliefs form the matrix of our functioning. Pema Chödrön, North American Buddhist nun and master teacher of meditation practice and theory, states unambiguously and succinctly, *"Mind is the source of everything,"* which is a fairly common philosophical and, currently, scientific notion (e.g., *What the Bleep Do We Know?* 2001). Unlike our *expectations*, which anticipate a specific material or spiritual outcome of our planned activities, and our *intentions*, which express our purpose for engaging in a particular act or acts, our core beliefs set the stage for all that we think, say, and do. Mahatma Gandhi (cited in Lipton, 2005, p.144) stated our beliefs become our thoughts which express as our words and actions. And our actions become our destiny.

All our self-talk and all our interactions reflect our core beliefs. As a former interpersonal communications colleague was fond of saying, *"You can not not communicate."* What we deeply communicate is what we believe about ourselves, others, and the world we share. Our silence, speech, voice, posture, facial expression, gestures, actions, vocabulary, and writings arise from our core beliefs. They express them. Underneath the words we use, underneath our manner of delivery of those words, underneath our particular bodily mannerisms, underneath our penchant for silence, reside our certainties, broadcasting our beliefs. That is why they so strongly affect our ability as therapists to help others. And that is why they deserve our keen attention.

We begin developing certainties early in life, some possibly prenatally, based on what we may hear, what we may feel, what we may sense, and our biology, family, society, and culture. They lead to our major decisions about what we believe to be true about ourselves, others, and the world outside ourselves. We make most of the far-reaching ones by the time we are six years old. After that, we add others that tend to reinforce the ones we already made. Eric Berne (1996) theorized that our certainties combine to orchestrate our entire life in the form of scripts (e.g., Steiner, 1990) which structure our every thought and act. The transactional analysis perspective underscores, *"The child is father to the man,"* as advised the poet Gerard Manley Hopkins. This notion succinctly summarizes the way most of us function. And that is not all good news. Living our life based on beliefs developed from the knowledge, experience, and cognitive capacities available to us as infants and young children inevitably leads to difficulty as we live them out as adolescents and adults. At 20 or 25 years of age and withdrawing, whining, blaming, and even throwing tantrums with loved ones or co-workers when we do not get to experience life on our terms reveals that we may be functionally no more than three years old emotionally and cognitively. That is the age at which we are certain we are the most important person in the universe, that we come first, and that others matter only insofar as they give us what we need and want, especially when we want it. How can we expect an adult functioning as an egocentric three-year-old to help establish a successful, healthy relationship with a partner or colleague especially when the partner or colleague is also three-years-old cognitively and emotionally? Or how can we expect to help create effective therapy relationships if we relate to clients, colleagues, students, employees, and the world around us as our three, or four, or five-year-old self?

Much of our difficulties arise not just from our outer circumstances, such as floods, war, pestilence, earthquakes, betrayal, theft of material goods, or from congenital or acquired personal challenges, such as albinism, diabetes, club foot, spinal bifida, head injury, AIDS, breast cancer, etc., but from our reactions to what we experience. To someone who knows us, we may seem to be living a wonderful life. We have a useful, respected career; a loving, responsible partner; adequate finances; physical attractiveness; and other accoutrements of our culture's norm for the successful individual. But when our experiences fail to jibe with our beliefs of what we should be experiencing, we may feel let down. Comparing our actual life with our idealized one, we may even conclude we have failed. We may become depressed, even suicidal. Rabbi Harold Kushner (2006) describes this not uncommon response to life as the "tyranny of the dream." For instance, if I have believed for some time I should be a painter with representation by prestigious New York City galleries and works purchased by notable museums, but I have difficulty getting my work accepted into local juried shows, I would eventually feel dejected and depressed. My friends may be impressed that I can create paintings. They even may purchase them for their own homes. But, because, my dream is to achieve greater renown than my friends' admiration for my work brings, and my dream remains the strongest influence on what I think, I dismiss their evaluation of my work and retain the notion to which my interpretation of the dream has lead, namely: I am a failure. Rabbi Kushner counsels people similarly crushed in the vise of their interpretation of core beliefs to use their current knowledge and cognitive ability to develop new, helpful beliefs grounded in current reality. This is not to say dreams need to be discarded if unrealized. They do need to be carefully considered when, after time, they appear impractical to determine whether or not and how to best realize them.

Our certainties not only influence our own feelings, thoughts, and behavior they also affect our biology. Recent research by Bruce Lipton (2005), cell biologist and early contributor to the emergent field of *epigenetics,* the study of the molecular mechanisms by which environment controls gene activity and the link between mind and matter, informs us that our core beliefs, not our DNA, determine our health and sense of well-being. He claims that, while environmental factors exert a stronger influence than DNA on individual cell behavior, *our beliefs about our environment override them both*, corroborating what Einstein avowed decades earlier: We live what we believe.

Lipton's and others' recent observations of the influence of belief on biology are in accord with the well-known *placebo effect* in clinical trials. During experiments assessing the effectiveness of pharmacological, surgical, or behavioral interventions, placebo's, which consist of the ingestion of inert substances, *pseudo* surgeries, or other treatments, such as unrelated forms of therapy, researchers frequently offer some patients placebo's as experimental controls to better evaluate the drug or procedure under question. In those instances, neither the practitioner nor the patient knows whether they have administered a placebo or the actual substance or procedure being assessed. Although placebos have no known value of themselves or relevance to the subjects' identified needs, analyses of their effects typically document they produce relief from suffering and even cures for diseases or maladies.

As a wizened, cherished relative once said to me, *"Placebo's are good medicine!"* Placebo's dramatic effects (e.g., Siegel, 1986) are thought to result from the belief of the clinician that he or she was doing something to help another, possibly combined with the belief of the patient that receiving treatment from an interested, attentive health care professional would be helpful. Nevertheless, for quite some time, health care researchers dismissed the placebo effect as simply an aberration. They seemed unwilling to consider the possibility that belief could affect behavior. But, with increasing reports of placebos' effectiveness and general interest in the effect of belief on our body systems (e.g., H. H. the Dalai Lama, 2005b), researchers, intrigued by the potential value of this low-cost, seemingly harmless manner of intervention, are directing more of their attention to the mechanism undergirding the placebo's effects.

Not only do our beliefs affect our own health, but, through our apparent mind-link connections with all around us (e.g., Jung, 1997: Sheldrake, 1982), they shape others' sense of their well-being as well (Goleman, 2006b). And, similarly, other peoples' beliefs influence our sense of peace and harmony. By adulthood, we've all had the experience of feeling calm in the presence of certain individuals and discomfort in the presence of others. A startling reaction I had to the person who would become my husband, then my ex-husband, remains an especially vivid example of this invisible linkage. Prior to the incident, I had had limited and impersonal contact with Frank through his position as statistical consultant to my advisor in the graduate program where I had recently enrolled. Even so, the limited exchanges we shared led me to consider him cold. Then, during the first research team meeting I attended as a newly appointed graduate research assistant to my faculty advisor, who directed the project, I experienced an unexpected depth to his coldness. Before Frank arrived and prior to the start of the formal meeting, those of us present had been enjoying light conversation. As he joined us in the room, almost all conversation stopped abruptly. And, within a second or so, the temperature of the air around me seemed to noticeably drop. I felt chilled on a comfortably warm September day.

I felt unnerved. There was no apparent physical explanation for what and how I felt. He did not open the door to enter the room; it had been open for some time. All windows were closed. I felt no draft. The coldness he exuded created the sensation of actual physical chilling of the air around me. I was frightened. I became stone still to be safe in the presence of something I experienced as deeply threatening. Yet, almost immediately, I discounted my frightening and objectively unsupportable feelings to adapt to this environment where only hard data seemed to matter. I shifted my concentration to the content and structure of the meeting and shoved my fear underground. And, within a year and one-half, I married the man because, like me, he was Jewish, and I could talk with him without hiding my intelligence! Had I heeded my initial, disturbing, and prescient impressions, rather than convincing myself they could not matter because they were unsupported by objective fact or logic (e.g., Gladwell, 2007), I would have avoided the prolonged intimate contact with him that hurt me deeply.

We all have experienced effects of others' presence subliminally. When we attend a party, go clubbing, or take quiet moments by ourselves at a coffee house to reflect on our day, we readily perceive whether we want to be there or not based on how we feel being in that space. If we feel comfortable, possibly energized, we probably stay for a while; if not, especially if we become tense or irritable, we may decide to leave as soon as possible. When we feel the need to escape from a social setting or a clinical experience, we need to place a premium on our own well-being and do that immediately, if not sooner, even though we may not at the time be able to readily verbalize why we feel as we do. We can reflect on why later when we are safely situated someplace else.

Years after I divorced my husband and worked as a senior therapist and team leader in an outpatient rehabilitation program for young, primarily male, adults who suffered traumatic brain injury, I relied on this yardstick to gauge my physical safety from moment-to-moment as I worked with clients. Because I had earned the reputation of working well with the most verbally and physically aggressive patients in the program, who also often happened to be the ones with extremely limited impulse control, they packed my caseload. I potentially was under siege from 8 am to 4:30 pm Monday through Friday, each week. Fortunately, by then, I had learned to tune into people fairly well and to trust what I felt to be true, even with these individuals, whose emotions could flip from one to another in an instant or less. Nevertheless, as a precaution, I routinely did the following: 1) I placed priority on maintaining a confident, stable, loving state-of-mind, especially during treatment; 2) I maintained a relatively consistent structure to our time together; and 3) I positioned myself so, if need be, I could exit first and safely from the small therapy room we shared. I never was hit or mistreated physically or verbally by any patient. In fact, the converse was true: Supervisors and fellow therapists marveled at the trust and love my patients showed me in so many concrete ways and the functional changes they achieved during our time together.

As we recognize how influential our beliefs are toward establishing and maintaining our own physical and emotional well-being and that of those around us whether expressed through words spoken (e.g., Telushkin, 1998) or written (e.g., Emoto, 2004) or radiated as thought and feeling (Goleman, 2006b), we can only conclude that establishing our own helpful belief system is in the best interest of us all in every way.

Transactional Analysis.

Studying Transactional Analysis (TA), which I began just prior to divorcing my husband, increased my awareness of the encompassing influence of our core beliefs, or certainties, on our thoughts, feelings, and behavior. TA (http://www.itaa-net.org/) considers the way we live our lives to be the expression of our core beliefs.

I became a trainee in the early '80's to develop a framework and a skill base from which to relate to clients themselves, not just their communication skills or lack of them. The alternative route to developing these key skills would have been to enroll in a university graduate program in counseling or psychology, which I did not believe would provide me the skill base I needed. I considered TA training, which encompassed approximately the same amount of calendar time, a more practical and direct exposure to a functional theory of personality and an exceptional opportunity to obtain the quality of supervised practice

I wanted as a therapist. Three additional reasons led me to choose this non-degree path to bolster my effectiveness as a clinician. First, TA skillfully uses linguistic structure and content to identify troublesome beliefs and behaviors and to help effect their change rather than pharmacological or electro-mechanical agents. Drawing on the strength of the recommended client-clinician relationship to provide a safe, reliable structure for change, the use of oral communications, or *transactions*, appeared meaningful and was comfortable territory for a speech-language pathologist, such as myself.

Second, TA places emphasis on action, not simply insight, to bring about desired change. Eric Berne (e.g., 1996) psychiatrist trained in psychoanalysis and founder of TA, widely communicated to patients, *"First change, and then we'll talk about it."* In fact, his over-riding goal for each patient was a 1-session cure. Like Eric Berne, I, too, wanted to help make therapy a short-term, healing experience. This commitment to achieving rapid and lasting change appealed greatly to me. I had witnessed the toll providing therapy year-after-year-after-year to the same clients, children and adults, enacted on both clients and therapists. Children who lisped, substituted "w" for "r.," or experienced stuttering problems often received therapy for two or more consecutive years without noticeably changing. When they eventually departed therapy, many felt sad and angry. They had become convinced they were different from their peers in unattractive ways that could not change. Similarly, I met adults in their 20's, 30's, and beyond disturbed that they continued to experience stuttering problems years after beginning treatment. They felt dismissive of speech therapy, which they felt did not deliver what it promised. Therapists also expressed anger and sadness when they ultimately had to face discharging clients who, after years of treatment, showed no appreciable gains, or who angrily and loudly departed believing speech therapy had failed them.

And Third, experienced TA therapists, certified by the International Transactional Analysis Association (www.itaa-net.org) as teachers of TA theory, practice, and principles, presented the focused curriculum geared to the interests and aptitudes of adult learners. For instance, the teacher/trainer in the first group I joined held a graduate degree in adult education. Most enrollee's I met were professionals providing human service, e.g., nurses, social workers, psychotherapists, clergy, accountants, teachers, etc. All of us sought refinement of our communication skills and a deeper, functional knowledge of human behavior and personality. We wanted to learn what to do and what not to do to become more effective in our work with clients and colleagues. But we did not want to just acquire more information; we wanted to learn how to change the way we were functioning. The TA training format structured, as it was, situated outside formal academic settings and simulating group treatment, the bedrock of TA, provided a comfortable, focused opportunity and personal feedback that helped us learn to identify core beliefs and to practice the communication skills needed to meet our goals.

UNCOVERING CORE BELIEFS

As enriching and useful as I have found learning to apply transactional analysis theory, principles, and practices to uncover core beliefs, I have come to prefer using two other approaches, equally helpful, but more direct and accessible. They are: *Asking and Answering Why?*, a form of personal journaling, and *Practicing Mindfulness Meditation*, which helps develop the mental focus required to uncover our core beliefs. As we identify our core beliefs, we have three choices: We can continue clinging to them and repeatedly suffer the discomfort, even suffering, they bring; we can modify them to make them relevant and helpful to our current circumstances; or we can replace them with considered, up-dated beliefs that lead to more harmonious living. These tools of deeper self-knowing, when applied with the sincere intent of greater self-knowledge, allow us to better ourselves and, as a result, become more helpful to others.

Asking and Answering *Why?*

As a graduate student at the University of Iowa, I learned a great deal about the effect of personal and group perceptions on human behavior in an enjoyable and participatory course entitled, General Semantics (Korzybski, 1955). General Semantics (GS) addresses the influence of language usage, our own and others', on our impression of ourselves, others, the world around us, and our place in it. The visiting instructor, Professor O.T. Bontrager, provided multiple opportunities in each class to question our individual core beliefs, or *certainties,* and several ongoing, semester-long projects to identify them. The most enduring experience for me was that of making a weekly entry in a personal journal. Each entry began by describing in detail a single incident we experienced that week that left us feeling frustrated, enraged, puzzled, or elated. The experiences detailed were of the *"I did not see it coming!"* variety. In TA terms, we described the *payoff* we experienced playing an interpersonal *game* (e.g., Berne, 1996), i.e., an unconscious, patterning of verbal and non-verbal transactions between two individuals arising from their core beliefs and habitual interaction styles. One minute, we enjoyed relative ease believing life was delivering what we hoped, or, at least, expected. The next moment we railed at our lot, disappointed, or, possibly, confused when it presented what we did not expect and, possibly, did not want.

All required that: 1) We did not hold ourselves, others, or circumstances responsible for the experience, recognizing it as the result, in part, of our own actions and 2) We write a detailed account of the specific actions of those involved in the particular set of circumstances and our thoughts and feelings throughout. 3) We analyze our involvement by repeatedly asking ourselves *"Why-questions,"* i.e., *Why did we do that?* and *Why did we feel that?* to reach the core belief or beliefs occasioning the behaviors and feelings under examination.

The following two examples encapsulate my use of this simple, powerful technique. The first summarizes my application of the tool to learn why I stuttered more severely than ever waiting for a root canal to begin. It is excerpted from a paper I presented at the 9th ISAD International Online Conference (Silverman, 2006c). The second, describes how I used the technique to learn why I accepted an adult for voice therapy, who I initially believed wan unmotivated to do the work necessary to achieve a clear, durable voice.

> *Example 1: The Need for Practice.* On a Friday afternoon, moments before 5 o'clock, I bit into a chocolate wafer and experienced the lingual surface of my right maxillary bicuspid fall away. I called my dentist's office immediately and learned, since I was experiencing no pain, I would have to wait until the coming Monday to be seen. That Monday the dentist informed me I needed a root canal. As I waited for the local anesthetic to take hold, my body could not have been more tense, overcome as I let myself be by the fear of facing what I was convinced would be improbable pain. Yet, attempting to divert my thinking to relate sensibly to my immediate environment and situation, I decided to ask the dentist sitting on my right a question about the pending procedure. I had had no experience or knowledge of what was involved. But my mind, continuing to concentrate on imminent pain, had no interest in functioning as an expressive language generator. I launched the string of words that was to have been the question but only sputtered, popping and spitting out sounds and syllables all over the place. Although the focus of my eyes was directed toward my lap, I sensed the sitting postures of the dentist on my right and the technician sitting on my left change from relaxed to stiff. Like me, they seemed to be barely breathing.
>
> While feeling astonished by the force of my stuttering and trying to stop, I noticed myself silently telling myself, *"Let it go. Let the stuttering be what it wants to be. Let it come out."* Receiving advice as I fiercely concentrated on suppressing and ending the stuttering and that advice in particular grabbed my attention. I refrained from further forcing and relaxed into the stuttering as I was learning to do through *shenpa* practice (Silverman, 2005), relinquishing the desire to escape from stuttering and the entire situation.
>
> Once the dentist began the root canal work, I hyperventilated. I also white-knuckled the chair arms, sweated big drops from my forehead, and screamed fluently.
>
> Later that evening with the anesthetic no longer in effect and feeling mentally composed, I decided to discover what was behind that surprising personal-worst/personal-best stuttering by Asking and Answering *Why?*

My first question to myself was: *Why did I stutter like that?* To which I responded, *I wasn't able to get my thoughts together. Why?* I asked. I answered: *I was fearful, so fearful I could neither think nor maintain necessary coordination between breathing and speaking.* To that, I asked *Why?* and answered, *Because I did not breathe evenly from my deep abdominal area to keep my mind calm and incisive; I let the fear overwhelm me, making my breathing shallow and irregular.* Again I asked myself *Why?* This time I answered, *Because I have not yet established the practice of even, deep abdominal breathing at all times.* And then I asked the *Why* that brought me to what I knew was the core belief underlying that unfamiliar, discomforting stuttering. because it drew out this response: *Because, when I heard of the practice, I understood why and how to do it. I felt I could easily perform it. And I thought I did not need to practice. I believed I could just "turn it on" when I felt strong emotion fill my mind. I did not fully take into account the speed and power of such emotion to disrupt the cognitive control of my behavior.* So, here it was, the core belief underlying this singular experience: *If I understand what I need to do, I can do it when I want to. I do not need to practice.* And me --- a therapist! I had to both laugh and wince at the truthfulness of that discovery.

That is the way I respond when I become aware of a core belief. I feel relief as though a weight encasing my body cracked, then dropped away. But the feeling usually is short-lived to be replaced with anger and shame that come from recognizing the difference between what I know about behaving and how I actually behaved. Finally, and usually quite soon afterward, I lighten up once more as I recognize the opportunity before me this realization has brought. That is when I resolve to substitute a more constructive belief for the one that led to pain.

This awareness has taken quite some time to achieve. Earlier, I abased myself whenever I failed to live up to my standards of what it meant to be perfect. The shame I felt that came from telling myself I was flawed kept me from active self-reflection. I simply did not want to collect more evidence suggesting I was imperfect. To believe I was would have threatened my very right to be. When I was able to accept I was no better nor no worse than any one I knew by occasionally failing to live up to personal standards, self-reflection became tolerable, even satisfying.

Had I continued castigating myself as ridiculous, stupid, and, even, hopeless for possessing personal imperfections as they revealed themselves through interpersonal-relationships, I would have suffered increasingly intense pain. So, by accepting I was no better or no worse than those I knew, I eventually realized I did not have to be perfect, *nor did they*. And that was when I realized that I also held the core belief *I must be perfect!* Instantaneously, it seems, I released it effortlessly wearing a broad smile. I have noticed experiencing such a moment of self-knowledge followed by self-acceptance releases energy that lightens the spirit and creates openness to further change, whatever that might be. *"You shall know the truth, and the truth shall set you free"* (John, 8:32).

Example 2:   Honor Intuition and Common Sense.   I first felt frightened when 52 year-old Abe abruptly abandoned voice therapy with me. As a young university professor in the mid- 1970's, I believed I should control those around me, at least students and clients. My failure to control the course of Abe's treatment forced me to face a vulnerability I did not want to touch, i.e., the recognition that I ultimately had no control over others, an understanding which took me many more years to appreciate and accept. But reflecting on the core belief that accounted for my rationale for accepting him as a client when my intuition and clinical knowledge suggested he had an extremely poor prognosis taught me even more about how I functioned as a professional and how I needed to change.

Abe had been successfully practicing trail law for many years, according to his account, until a surgical mishap allegedly damaged his voice. He approached me as a speech-pathologist and university professor referred to him by staff at The Mayo Clinic. They suggested he consult with me, a speech pathologist residing where he lived, as a therapist who might be able to help him recover a serviceable voice and return to work.

I did not trust Abe's motivation for seeking help. While he expressed a passion for trial work despite an anxiety about an uncertain yet probable reduced income should he continue his practice, I did not believe he wanted to resume working. He announced, with a fierce display of righteous anger, that he had begun malpractice litigation against the anesthesiologist who had performed what he considered the ill-fated intubation that led to his now weak, raspy, poorly sustainable voice. Perhaps, it was that declaration that made me suspicious. But, even if I had not heard the words he uttered and only witnessed his facial expression, particularly the look that emanated from his eyes, I would have been unconvinced that recovering his pre-operative voice was what he wanted. I felt he viewed his current happenstance as an opportunity to retire early from trial work in a financially comfortable style, and I believed he was seeking treatment, which he expected to fail, only to bolster his claim that his present voice would be his permanent one.

I, nevertheless, accepted him as a client because he was my first referral from The Mayo Clinic, which provided copies of his medical records indicating he, indeed, had experienced a protracted period of intubation related to his dysphonia, and I hoped for subsequent referrals from them. And I was an avowed Rescuer (Please See Chapter 2) tantalized by the opportunity of working with such a seemingly sympathetic client.

Within the first treatment session, I was convinced my intuition concerning his motivation and intent was accurate. His condescending, almost mocking, responses to requests to perform vocal tasks, which he performed with consistently forced whispers followed by aggressive "I told you so" smirks, did not bode well for a clinically successful outcome. During the fourth session, which I recorded as I had all previous ones, I engaged him in a conversation concerning a topic of high interest to him. As he spoke with animation, even fervor, his voice became normal in less than a minute or so, with no trace of effort or breathiness. As soon as he realized he had produced a clear, appropriately loud voice, and sustained it he abruptly stopped speaking. I, elated we now had indisputable evidence he might recapture his pre-operative, or at least a serviceable, voice, thought he would feel similarly. He did not. He appeared stunned, shocked, even shrunken and became uncharacteristically subdued throughout the remainder of the session. At the conclusion, he rushed from the room contrary to his usual, cheery departures.

He never returned, nor did he call to explain why. But I did receive a phone call from the psychologist helping him deal with the grief and loss issues he said he felt as a result of his altered voice. The psychologist wanted to hear the tape segment which Abe told him indicated I thought demonstrated he had the capacity to produce a serviceable voice. We arranged to meet several days later. When he, too, heard the sample he looked as stunned and as sickened as Abe and raced for the door. I never saw or head from either one again.

This clinical experience was a first for me. Never before had I disregarded a strong intuitive feeling about a pending client. I wanted to understand why. So, I made the time to begin *Asking and Answering Why*. As usual, I started by secluding myself to secure necessary privacy. Then I asked myself, *Why did I rebel against my intuition to take on a client evincing no evidence of wanting to participate in treatment to change?* To which I replied after much thought, *Because I wanted the challenge of besting this arrogant, little person who thinks he can beat the system and me. Why? Because I wanted the satisfaction of seeing him squirm when he knew he was beaten. Why did I need to do that?* And my reply leading directly to the core belief behind my reason for accepting him as a client was: *I need to prove myself as competent and strong even if that comes across as cruel.* My core belief: I need to be right! Being right justifies my existence, it seems, and I know why. That belief arose when I was three, and for reasons unrelated to this situation. What does require comment, though, is that I recognized this core belief not only affected my clinical-decision making for Abe, but, in all likelihood, affected how I related to all potential and actual clients and, no doubt, caregivers, colleagues, and students. And, so, I resolved to release that firmly entrenched, troublesome belief. Training in transactional analysis helped by introducing the concept of *contracting,* a process undertaken when initiating treatment and, often, throughout its course. The key tenet underlying contracting, relates to framing clinical interactions with others as mutually collaborative events (e.g., Berne, 1977).

A Note About the Process

I find the process of uncovering core beliefs more effective when approached as a journaling task rather than speaking out loud to myself or silently thinking. Most of us are more accustomed to speaking and thinking than writing about our personal concerns, so writing slows us down. That change in pace can help heighten our perceptiveness. Also, as we consider the words we are about to write or the ones we have written, we find that writing demands greater truthfulness than does our usual, often, glib speech, to help us more easily reach the core (Sarton, 1992). For instance, my tendency is to say *"I don't know."* When, talking to myself and asking, *"Why?"* I would not enter that response into a journal because reading those words on a computer screen or on a page of the journal would tell me I am resisting completing the necessary detective work fearful as I am of what I might discover. Recognizing that is true makes me determined to screw up my courage and dig deep. That is the power of writing.

Practicing Mindfulness

> *"Mr. Duffy"... lived a short distance from his body... "*
>
> --- James Joyce, *The Dubliners*

Like Mr. Duffy we, too, are rarely present. We seem to be where we are, but mentally, we are someplace else. We may be sitting on a park bench on a beautiful sunny day, but we don't feel the cool breezes move across our face and arms. We don't hear the sweet notes of a robin's song. We don't see the dogs frolicking on the empty baseball diamond across the way. We don't experience the fragrance of the extravagant lilac blooms behind us. Instead, we worry, or plan, or chat on our cell phone to avoid the anxious feeling that arrives when we feel alone We attend our son's soccer game, but we miss watching him block an opponent's kick because we were text messaging at the time. We sit on the sofa cuddled next to our partner at the end of a hectic day to watch a DVD, but, mentally, we are rehearsing what we will say to our neighbor tomorrow about the block party scheduled for next weekend. And, we drive to work at 70 miles per hour on the expressway while drinking coffee, putting on makeup, making and taking calls, or planning what we will do when we get there! We rarely focus on being where we are and, in so doing, risk losing our precious lives.

Mostly, we act mindlessly (e.g., Langer, 1989). I remember, more than once, finding my ex-husband standing in the pantry of our house holding an opened jar of peanut butter and sucking a glob of it from his right index finger. Startled, as if suddenly waking from a dream when he noticed me staring at him, he would utter quietly, *"I don't know how I got here."* I was sure he did not. Lost in thought almost all the time, he behaved like the archetypal, absent-minded professor. Perhaps he thought being an actual professor required that he behave in an absented-minded way. Of course, I never experienced any lapses in attention!

Practicing mindfulness meditation (e.g., Hanh, 2004: Kabat-Zinn, 2006; 2005) trains our minds to be present (e.g., Silverman, 2005; Silverman, 2003d) so that we are more aware of what we are thinking, feeling, saying, and doing at the moment. Being mindful, unlike fear-based vigilance, helps open us to the world. Being mindful allows us to be present and to encourage those around us to be present as well and helps us develop deeper insight into events and circumstances. That gives us great leverage to put into place new beliefs and behaviors.

Being present also allows us to monitor our almost constant *internal dialogue*. Otherwise, we may unwittingly talk to ourselves the way our abusive caregivers did and maintain our *status quo* or lose ground by strengthening destructive habits, instead of believing and behaving as we wish. For instance, my mindless internal dialogue sounds like tape recordings of my late father's and late stepmother's abusive behavior toward me. My father called me, *"The Big Dummy."* Whenever he thought I failed to notice someone's apparently devious inclinations, he screamed, *"All you know is book knowledge, 'You Big Dummy.'"* Sometimes, when I entered a room, he would eye me with a mixed look of amusement and disdain and snarl, *"There's 'The Big Dummy.' Look at 'The Big Dummy.'"* Before I was 12, I was referring to myself as *"The Big Dummy"* whenever I behaved in a manner I felt was naïve, and I felt just as angry toward myself and, then, hurt as if my father, who expected me to live by standards he alluded to but failed to take the time to teach, slammed that ugly label on me. My stepmother referred to me as, *"Big Fat Tub of Lard."* I shortened that into, *"I'm fat,"* an appellation by which I denigrated myself for decades. When I began practicing mindfulness meditation and attending to my internal dialogue, I realized I was referring to myself, someone who wore a size 8 or10 pants or dress, as fat. With that realization, I held a distorted view of my attractive, useful, physical body. My body image and my self image, severely distorted by my long-term, false internal dialogue required major overhauls. Being mindful of what I was saying to myself about myself helped me stop that form of self-denigration.

Meditation practices that help develop and build on mindfulness include Insight Meditation (e.g., Kornfield, 2001, 1998; Salzberg and Goldstein, 2002), *Shenpa* Practice (e.g., Chödrön, 2005b; Silverman, 2005), and *Tonglen* Meditation (Chödrön, 2005b). Insight Meditation focuses on looking deeply into circumstances and events to develop understanding including he deepest form of understanding, or *vipassana. Shenpa* Practice, helps break habitual thought and behavior patterns such as those associated with stuttering problems (Silverman, 2005). And *Tonglen* Meditation develops and engages compassion for ourselves and others. Like the process of *Asking WHY?* Tonglen Meditation uses our unpleasant experiences to deepen our self-awareness, compassion toward self and others, and our membership in the human community, and, unlike *Asking WHY?*, it also uses our pleasant experiences to the same ends.

A practice that utilizes both imagery and sound combined, i.e., Tibetan sound healing from the ancient *Bön* Buddhist tradition (e.g., Wanygal, 2006), uses the controlled application of the mind to restore and enhance mental and physical well-being. While, this may not be a meditation form in a purist sense, the practice does benefit from and enlarge an established meditation practice. I have found it quite helpful in creating mental focus and clarity.

Meditation (e.g., Fontana, 1999), an ancient, natural process, has become a mainstream activity in the United States. Approximately 10 million Americans, children and adults, practice some form of meditation daily. We may practice to become more relaxed, more in touch and in partnership with our physical body, more aware of and involved with the activity of our mind, and more involved in our faith experience. We may adopt a method associated with practices of the Christian, Judaic, Islamic, Native American or other sacred traditions or from among methods bearing no direct connection to religious practices, for example, mindfulness based stress reduction (MBSR) (Kabat-Zinn, 2006, 2005). But for the practice to infuse daily life with serenity, compassion, and deep understanding these fruits of a meditation practice need to be applied to everyday life.

The selection of medication practices to cultivate is vast and includes many forms of sitting meditation and walking meditation. For those of us who want to become who we wish to be, methods that cultivate mindfulness and concentration are most helpful. When we learn to live in the present, rather than in the past or future, and attend to our momentary thoughts, feelings, and bodily sensations, we have real opportunity to change our beliefs and behaviors as we will. As the humor therapist, Loretta La Roche (2002) reminds us: *"The past is history. The future is a mystery. Now is a gift. That's why it's called The Present."*

Other Tools. I also have found working with archetypes (e.g., Myss, 2002a), dreams analysis (e.g., Bosnak, 1986), journaling (e.g., Progoff, 1983), and narrative medicine principles and practices (Charon, 2006), which I co-opted as a practice I labeled narrative speech pathology (Silverman, 2004), helpful in uncovering my core beliefs, and so have others. But, for me, practicing mindfulness makes my use of the other methods more effective. By learning to be mindful, I can calm and stabilize my mind to reach the concentration level needed for steady penetration into the subconscious and to reach my unconscious as well as the collective unconscious (e.g., Jung, 1997) where individual and primal core beliefs reside.

CORE BELIEFS AND PROFESSED BELIEFS

Our core beliefs, or *certainties*, not necessarily our professed ones, help define who we think we are, what we experience, and how we behave. A while ago, someone I knew quite well offered me what she hoped I would accept as high praise or, possibly, flattery, when she told me, *"I never knew anyone who so completely lives their beliefs as you do."* I did not respond quite as she expected in either case. I did not smile or express any gratitude for her supposed compliment. Instead, I responded tartly, *"Everyone lives their beliefs."* She scowled. She appeared angered by my unwillingness to be manipulated and, possibly, by my insinuation that she did not live the beliefs she professed to value. A guarded, yet superficially charming person to those susceptible to personal flattery, who believed she had the skill to convince others to accept at face value what she chose to say about herself and others, she did not want to hear that someone recognized that the personal image she cultivated differed vastly from the image she gave off. By appearing to praise me as she did, she implied she does not think well of those and, possibly, herself who do not live according to their professed values. Yet, to the time of her death, she made no recognizable effort to change. She valued personal popularity possibly more than any other individual accomplishment. That belief lead her to openly express beliefs she thought may impress others, even when the way she lived contradicted what she said. For instance, she announced to people she believed would be impressed by knowing she followed a vegetarian diet that she was a vegetarian, but she publicly ate meat when she believed being known as a vegetarian might cause someone to devalue her in some way. One of her core beliefs seemed to be: *My words speak louder than my actions.* That was how she lived. And those who knew her readily recognized that and referred to her as phony because they knew, as do you and I, that actions speak louder than words.

We label those who say they live one way but appear to live just the opposite, hypocrite. And, at one time or another, most of us may have deliberately behaved as one when our goal, like hers, was to make a favorable impression or to just get by in a difficult situation, such as, pretending to like a client or caregiver we found unattractive in one way or another but did not want to fully admit that fact to ourselves or to directly address it. Such a not uncommon scenario could arise from the core belief, *I Have To Be*

Accommodating to All My Clients All The Time Even If That Means Living A Lie. Not being completely honest with ourselves by recognizing what we feel and believe and directly addressing those realities is to greatly reduce our professional effectiveness because most clients will detect any incongruence between how we relate to them and how we seem to feel about them. When they perceive discontinuity between our beliefs and behaviors, they will consider us untrustworthy.

Being inauthentic also reduces our own satisfaction with our work. Believing one way and behaving another way takes much more energy than being authentic. That, of itself, increases our stress and fatigue and fortifies the barrier between us and our clients from our inauthenticity because it discourages the heartfelt communication that would energize us. Our clients, especially young children, know they can relate to us when we are present and that they can not when are emotionally absent. That is when they turn away, perhaps never to fully return.

There are times, though, when we may seem to be living hypocritically when, in fact, we are in process of shifting from living an unhelpful belief to a helpful one we profess to value. That process takes some time before it is complete, and, until then, we behave inconsistently. For instance, I believe I should practice patience, and, "Why not?" That's what mature people do. Taking time to make a considered response to what life brings instead of reacting, usually emotionally, from incomplete information, to eventually suffer the painful consequences that brings benefits us all. Allowing life to unfold in its own time and way rather than forcing an outcome avert what often is unnecessary unpleasantness we, otherwise, inadvertently inflict ourselves and on others. But being patient has been quite difficult for me since I was very young. An aunt, my mother's sister, enjoyed teasing the adult me by saying sing-song, *"I'm ready; I'm waiting!"* when she thought I was being impatient. She did that because she insisted that was what I chanted before mealtime when I was three. Apparently, as soon as I saw the table had been set, I climbed onto a chair at the table and repeated, *"I'm ready. I'm waiting." u*ntil someone found a way to di*stract me.* Telling me, *"You have to wait; dinner (or breakfast or lunch) is not ready yet."* never worked. So they learned not to set the table until the moment they were ready to serve the meal.

Well, I believe I have made some progress shifting from believing *"I should receive what I want when I want it"* to *"I will have what I need when I need it."* since I made living patiently a distinct personal goal twenty years ago. Among the many signposts of how I have changed are: I now can sit behind the steering wheel of my car when stuck in traffic without grimacing or thinking many angry thoughts. I can coax my dog off the bed when I want to make it rather than angrily and repeatedly shouting, "OFF!" while tugging at the bedding until he jumps out of bed. And I can wait to make a trip to buy groceries until I actually need an item or items instead of using shopping as an excuse to amuse myself. But, after 20 years, I am not yet consistently patient. That was apparent while posing for a photographer last week for a casual head shot needed to accompany an article I wrote. The photographer agreed to shoot in my well-planted front yard where I am at ease, and she seemed to genuinely care about meeting the editorial requirements. But it was a windy, unusually chilly, October day and a day when my back hurt. After standing where she placed me here and then there as she searched for a location to best accommodate the changing sunlight as it filtered through the clouds then went direct when they rolled away, I developed a severe case of *blinkitis.* That meant she took many more exposures than would otherwise have been taken. I wanted this process, which I was certain would produce an image of an irritated woman I really did not want to share with my colleagues, to end quickly. With that irritation that impatience brought oozing from my voice, I asked how much longer she expected to continue. She tartly replied, *"Until I get the image I want."* I knew from her words, her tone of voice, and her posture, that is exactly how long she would take. Rather than being pleased and thankful I had selected such a conscientious professional for the job, I focused on my feelings of discomfort which naturally magnified them. That led to my increased impatience and decreased cooperation. Instead of communicating meaningfully with the camera lens, I mentally withdrew from the active process to silently worry about how the images she captured would represent me to colleagues. Fortunately, we were able to select one image reflecting relatively few facial clues of impatience and irritation. That experience and the unmistakable visual evidence of my impatience with the photographer reminded me I still do not always act as I profess I wish to act.

Am I behaving like a hypocrite? No. I am someone in transition, and, in that process, the older, more habituated belief and related behavioral expressions trump the newer, more fragile belief-behavior link, especially when anxious. This is what we face personally and what our clients also experience when we commit to changing what we believe. This is where patience mixed with perseverance becomes essential. We do not know how long it will take us to fully change into behaving consistently as we wish, but we do know that we probably will not do so unless we practice the right behavior and the right self-talk for as long as it takes.

What follows is a short vignette highlighting the behavior of an adult client who refused to change how she spoke but professed, through her faithful attendance at a support group for adults that was what she wanted to do.

> *Marcella.* When I was an undergraduate enrolled in a course on stuttering, the instructor invited a few of us at a time to attend meetings of the support group she facilitated for adults with stuttering problems. The members seemed enthusiastic about our attendance and the opportunity to personally teach students about the real-life experience of living with a stuttering problem. The evening I attended one group member, at the instructor's request, demonstrated each of the various Van Riper speech control techniques we had been studying. Marcella, who previously had stuttered that evening forcing out almost every word,

was completely fluent during her demonstration. That amazing effect on her speech and confidence was no different than if a magician had pointed his wand at her and said, *"Hocus-Pocus, Abracadabra Marcella, You are completely fluent!"* Afterward one of us asked her why she did not use the techniques all the time. Smiling, she answered, *"Because they don't feel natural."*

Perhaps Marcella did not practice speaking with the techniques long enough and appropriately enough for them to "feel natural" because she really did not want to change (Myss, 1997; Silverman, 2007a). I believe she did not want to change. I later learned she, someone in her late 30's, had held the same job, lived in the same apartment, engaged in the same social activities, and maintained the same circle of friends for most of her adult life. Therapy in this particular milieu, which she attended for many years, fit snuggly into her circumscribed life as a social event inadvertently reinforcing sameness. Marcella wanted to maintain her *status quo.* She seemed to believe, *It's safest to stay with what you know. You don't know what will happen if you change.* And with that certainty in place she would not and could not change how she spoke. And neither could anyone else.

We need always to be alert when someone requests treatment as to whether they are seeking treatment to satisfy someone else's needs or whether they genuinely wish to change.

THE CHALLENGE OF DESIRED PERSONAL CHANGE

Change is certain. Nothing stays the same.

Cliché? Yes, and, oh, so true! Today we like mocha lattes. Yesterday we preferred cherry coke. This season we decided to root for the Green Bay Packers. Last year we were Jets fans. Now we're happily dating laid-back Sam. Last week we paired with Funky Jim. Like everyone and everything else, we change from moment to moment physically and mentally and emotionally as well, if we allow ourselves to do that. Consider our mammoth change from fetus, to infant, to toddler, to child, to adolescent, to adult. And we are not done. Change is what we are about, and we need to be smart about it. The best use of our time is to manage change well, our own and our clients'. While we have some latitude to choreograph our physical metamorphosis and to orchestrate our involvement with others and even, to some extent, our mental agility, we can always alter our beliefs until the very end. That is why some religions encourage death-bed confessions and conversions.

Changing Our Beliefs to Change Our Behavior

Knowing that changing our beliefs changes our lives, we can replace our limiting beliefs with helpful ones when we want to change our lives for the better. If we do not want to change our lives, we will find all sorts of reasons not to change our beliefs despite insisting change is what we want. Recall Marcella: She insisted she wanted to be free of her stuttering problem. That was why she regularly attended individual and group therapy sessions. That was why she learned each of the various speech controls therapists introduced to her. And that was why she did not use them to permanently change the way she spoke. Deep down, she knew if she did, she could no longer continue living life as she knew it. She would have to contend with changes she could not fully foresee and, possibly, not control. Without severely stuttered speech as an excuse, she would need to actively seek the management position she said she desired because she stuttered and to do the dating to find the partner she claimed she wanted. And without severely stuttered speech, she would no longer have the basis for feeling special as she did, for instance, by participating in the support group where she experienced deep satisfaction from helping instruct future speech therapists about stuttering, even though feeling special by having a severe stutter also brought feelings of shame, embarrassment, fear, and isolation. That was the price she was willing to pay to feel special, a feeling most of us desire. So, she made the choice to continue to stutter severely so she could continue to live the life she knew rather than adopting the belief that *Taking Considered Risks Can Bring Great Personal Rewards.* In this way, she is like so many of us, even the fictional townspeople of European and Chinese folklore, who, given the chance to exchange their individual burdens for another's, all chose to keep their own. Hateful as they considered their own burdens to be, they preferred what they knew to what they did not, even though what was unknown to them eventually might have been more to their liking.

Changing our core beliefs and, by so doing, changing our lives is one of the most difficult tasks we can assume (Das, 2003). After all, as history and biographies convincingly reveal, our core beliefs are what we are willing to live for and die for and, if need be, kill for. Only when we become distraught enough, desperate enough, or courageous enough will we make the effort to change what we deeply believe. In a simplistic way, getting started changing our beliefs mirrors getting started clearing out our clothes closets. Letting go of outmoded and outgrown wardrobe pieces along with the memories and self-concepts attached to them can be frightening. We feel doing so eliminates some of who we are. We identify with our apparel and accessories because they hold memories of times, pleasant and unpleasant, spent with people important to us and because, as they helped us project an element of our *persona* into the world, we treasure them as reminders of what we have accomplished. Relinquishing these items can generate much anxiety for us because we feel we are losing a part of ourselves. That is why managing our closets, and our clutter in general, can be a task we choose to defer even though we know deciding which skirts, tops, dresses, pants, sweaters, shoes, boots, and accessories meet our present needs and discarding those which do not frees up personal space while helping us live less hassled lives.

We put off the job until wrestling with our over-stuffed closet becomes more unpleasant than what we expect may be involved refreshing it. When we tire of taking too long to locate particular pieces or smoothing out crumpled ones, we finally may start cleaning. Similarly, when we look into our mental storehouses for knowledge and ideas to bring more satisfaction into our life and find it stuffed with unused and outworn beliefs and practices from we gleaned from books, articles, coursework, conferences, inservices, and workshops, that we now realize runs counter to what we consider necessary and helpful, we need to update the contents. Taking the time and making the effort to discard beliefs and practices that offer no solution to current dilemmas and may create additional ones seems a smart choice.

Changing Our Behavior to Change Our Beliefs

Sometimes, the easiest way to introduce helpful beliefs into our lives is to first change our behavior (Weil, 1995) to conform to what our target beliefs suggest. For example, Shakyamuni Buddha, the historical Buddha, exhorted those attracted to his teachings to test them before adopting them. An exemplar teacher, the Buddha encouraged individuals to rely on direct, personal experience to draw their own conclusions about how to live, using his teaching as a guide, not a mandate. Then, if they found they preferred living according to his teaching, to adopt those beliefs. Similarly, if we cling to the belief *I Can't Lose Weight and Keep It Off* from our many failed experiences dieting, we may want to test that belief. if our desire to be healthier and attractive has been kindled or re-kindled by reports that ordinary people have achieve desired outcomes by living a healthy lifestyle. Noting their enthusiasm, we take up the same practices. We may then discover another limiting belief to test: *I Can't Take Time for Myself Because I'm Not Worth it*. Making the commitment to eat healthfully and to exercise appropriately and incorporate those goals into our daily lives and experiencing weight loss and increased energy, we may then find we can substitute the positive belief, *I Can Lose Weight and Keep It Off When I Live a Healthy Lifestyle*, for the old, limiting one that kept us fat and exhausted, after proving to ourselves that we can.

Application to Speech-Language Pathology. Changing behavior to change beliefs is a common feature of speech therapy with those who have stuttering problems or voice problems. For example, we often begin by collaborating with clients to outline a program of behavioral change for them to undertake for which we offer direction and encouragement. We rarely concentrate initially on helping clients acquire insight to facilitate change; we concentrate on helping them to establish useful behavior to facilitate lasting change. Once any of us begin to change, we become encouraged to believe we can continue until we reach our ultimate goal, as we apply the necessary endurance bolstered through ongoing , constructive self-talk. This is the approach Eric Berne, founder of transactional analysis (1996), directed toward patients with whom he worked, and the way Chasidic rabbis of Eastern Europe aided depressed community members. When the individuals in need became more satisfied with their lives after changing their behaviors, these facilitators became willing to discuss personal beliefs. *Change First, Talk About It Later* was their *leitmotif*.

Balance

From my experience, change requires a combination of insight and action throughout. Sometimes, changing behavior begins after a glimmer of insight suggests desired change is possible. For instance several decades ago, I began a successful program of significant weight loss, despite having been convinced by my stepmother I would be fat for as long as I lived. But when, during an annual physical examination, an internist convinced me I owed it to myself, a young and attractive woman, to loose my extra poundage and enjoy life while I could, I began to believe I could become trim and fit. His suggestion, so sincere, so logical, and so unsolicited fatally cracked my long-held belief, *I Will Always Be Fat*. On the spot, I began to think, *"I can loose weight. I should loose weight. He believes I can do it. I think I can."* As I scrupulously followed the advice in the pamphlet he offered me that day and began losing the weight I thought was mine to drag around forever, my false belief crumbled. My new behavior created a new belief: *I Can Weigh The Right Weight for Me*. So, the insight he stimulated started a process of phenomenal weight loss for me and, not incidentally, an identical focus in my work with others. Like him, my primary goal is to be compassionate, encouraging, and helpful. I am *paying it forward*!

I also accomplished another major change, quitting smoking, by first changing my belief. When I was a college senior, the U.S. Surgeon General's Report implicated cigarette smoking as a serious health hazard. By then, I smoked about one pack each day, and I was beginning to suspect that I was not doing myself any good by doing that. While I had not previously considered I might be harming myself by smoking, I was concerned that I was smoking too much. Without using the word *addict* to describe my smoking behavior, I was fearful I had become one. That notion was extremely disturbing. I had always needed to be free of any restriction on my personal freedom. I did not want to be controlled by needing to smoke. So I decided to stop. A friend and I decided to quit together to provide each other with the moral support we were sure we would need. Her resolve lasted a few hours, mine about a day. Each of us independently convinced ourselves quitting was too hard for us.

Several years later, as a graduate student writing my dissertation and smoking two packs of cigarettes daily, I knew I had to quit. I had a smoking related chronic cough that daily expelled plugs of thick, yellowish phlegm from my lungs and trachea. My tongue tip felt raw. And I detested feeling like a slave to this expensive, now unfulfilling, habit. Yet I knew I could not yet successfully handle the stress of ending the habit while stressed by the demands of graduate work. So I promised myself I would quit the day after my final oral defense of my dissertation. And I did! That was 40 years ago, and I have not smoked anything since. What I had learned about the health-related dangers of smoking from medical reports and from my personal experience living with the increasingly distressing habit combined irrefutably to convince me quitting was in my best interest. To do that, I first discarded my belief, *I Can Do What I Want With My Body Because I'm Invulnerable*, to replace it with a saner one, *I Must Take Good Care of My Precious Body*, to quit smoking. So, in my experience, desired change can be accomplished by first changing behavior to test a related belief that is beginning to seem false or by first discarding an apparent false belief to replace it with an acceptable, helpful one and the behaviors it engenders..

When I am clear in my mind what it is I wish to change and why, then I can visualize the outcome of my efforts and direct them toward realizing that change. For instance, when I committed to stopping smoking, I visualized myself at the conclusion of the process as smiling, cough-free, and radiant. That image propelled me forward in all my efforts to change my lifestyle from smoker to nonsmoker. Acting with concentration and focus, we keep our eyes on the prize and direct our efforts toward achieving it. That way we can eventually claim it.

MANAGING DESIRED PERSONAL CHANGE

To best manage our personal change, we need to: Make time for ongoing self-reflection (e.g., Silverman, 2008) and relate to ourselves with kindness and compassion.

Ongoing Self-Reflection.

Others' lives are so intriguing! Following the lives of celebrities almost seems an obsession. We want to know where they party and with whom, where they vacation and with whom, where they live and with whom, where they shop and what they buy, and so on. And we similarly observe co-workers, neighbors, family members, and partners. We take note of our children's friends, which is necessary to a point, for their safety. But we spend little, if any, time getting to know our true selves. We say we are too busy. We have jobs, family, and community responsibilities to meet that leave us little to no time to reflect on our lives. Yet, each day, we watch several hours of television, play podcasts, watch DVD's, listen to music, read magazines and newspapers, gossip with family and friends, walk the dog, exercise, and shop. If we find ourselves momentarily quiet and alone, we become edgy. We feel uncomfortable with the sudden silence and inactivity. We quickly find something to eat or to do to relieve our anxiety. Nothing, it seems, frightens us more than being alone (e.g., Myss, 2002c). Maybe that is because, when we are alone, we know we may become reacquainted with the submerged pain we carry, and we fear touching it may overwhelm us.

I remember those apprehensions so well. It was not until 1981, when a friend, a nun, who usually spoke to me with great directness said, *"You have to go through the pain."* Hearing those words and noting her fierce facial expression as she seemed to hurl them at me was not what I wanted to hear. I did not want to *"go through the pain"* again. Once had been enough. Thank you! But Sr. Joan challenged me to go through it to put it behind me. Dragging it around was dragging me down. I was sick with colds and flu more often than those around me, and I was joyless almost all the time because so much of my vital energy was wastefully spent running from my unresolved feelings.

Not immediately, but after a while, I followed her advice. I began to acknowledge individual hurts and pains from near or far away as they presented themselves during meditation, the only time I was quiet enough to consciously detect their presence in my mind or in my body. Slowly, I learned to acknowledge these feelings as painful as they were when fresh, to work with them, and to finally resolve them. After a while, I noticed something quite remarkable happening: I was growing stronger. I became more confident in my ability to speak and to make my way in this world. I was joyful on occasion. And I was more understanding of those I knew and encountered and of myself. Unfortunately, I still am sick more often than I think someone living as healthful a lifestyle as I do should be, but I am confident even that matter will resolve itself.

I have learned that when we take time as adults to know ourselves, we become able to live our lives as well as we might. And we become able to be as helpful to others as we might. Spending as few as 10 or even 5 minutes of quiet time alone in daily prayer, meditation, reflection, contemplation, and/or journaling can help us know and be ourselves. If we do not help ourselves, not even the Buddha's (Kongtrul, 2006) nor, possibly, God, can help, since, as President John Fitzgerald Kennedy stated in his inaugural address, *"Here on earth, God's work is truly our own."*

Of course, making the effort to know ourselves does not mean we only will discover unhelpful behaviors to change. We may recognize previously undetected talents and abilities. For example, someone using journaling as a self-reflection tool may discover a talent as a writer of prose or poetry. Someone else may recall how much they enjoyed drawing as a child and decide to build on that interest. Another may recall the pleasure of making music by playing the piano and resume practicing. Someone else may discover their sense of humor and find they enjoy taking the stage at the local comedy club open mike night, and so on. Uncovering talents and abilities and integrating them into the fullness of our being is another benefit of self-reflection.

Relating with Kindness and Compassion

Many of us resolve to change only after believing we have failed in an intimate relationship, at our profession, or in some other way. When we use personal failure as motivation to change, we often begin the process feeling angry at ourselves, especially if we experienced our caregivers relate to us with anger when we irritated them. We also may start out shamed and embarrassed because that was our reaction to feeling like a failure when we were young. If we step back to observe how relating to ourselves so harshly affects us physically and emotionally, we will notice we become constricted and draw ourselves tightly inward. By so doing, we thwart, rather than nourish, our effort to cultivate new, constructive thought-behavior sets. We stunt our own growth. To change as we wish, we need to relate to ourselves with kindness, warmth, and compassion throughout the process even, and especially, when we fail to measure up to our own or anyone else's expectations. In this way, we grow like a flower encouraged by the sun's warming rays to open our petals and bloom rather than shrivel and decay as we would after being tinged by frost..

Learning to relate kindly to ourselves after years, possibly decades, of self-denigration is a process for which we need reminders from time-to-time. Pema Chödrön, North American Buddhist nun and master meditation teacher, generously shared a challenge she experienced during a week-long retreat when she, too, needed a reminder to be kind to herself (Chödrön, 2005b; Silverman, 2006c).

> Pema found herself experiencing deep, wordless anxiety daily while meditating. As she had learned, she resolved to remain present with the feeling, neither denying nor suppressing it. She also applied various techniques to soften and melt it away. But the feeling persisted. After some time, she presented this, to her, troubling circumstance to her teacher, Dzigar Kongtrul Rinpche, for resolution. He reported he himself had had such an experience that lasted several moths and disclosed that, for him, it had been a good teacher. Encouraged that the feeling would eventually dissolve, she continued working to release the feeling, but still it persisted. Later, when her teacher joined her during meditation, he announced, *"Oh, I know that feeling. That's the Dakini Bliss!"*
>
> *"Dakini Bliss?"* Pema vocalized excitedly. *"Oh, wow! Right! The feeling does have the intensity of bliss,"* she rhapsodized. Once she believed she was experiencing something special, she felt special. And she became eager to embrace the feeling, to welcome it as a valued guest. But it was gone and did not return.

Pema understood why: She knew surrendering to what seems undesirable dissolves the feeling and relating to ourselves with warmth and kindness helps us do that. Before her teacher intervened, she considered being unable to remove the anxiety as a personal failure. And because she believed she was failing, she struggled against further failure. Her struggling distracted her from direct experience of the feeling and increased her concern about personal worthiness. When her teacher reframed her discomforting experience as desirable,

Pema re-imaged it as well. In the light of his words, she then considered herself a success, not a failure. Immediately, she changed the way she responded. She no longer felt shame, guilt, impatience, and, possibly, anger because of her presumed failure. Instead, she enjoyed feeling victorious. She relaxed. She ceased struggling. Her anxiety disappeared.

Like Pema, we, too, encounter situations that try us by tempting us to struggle against ourselves and, perhaps, conclude we failed. We may react as she by struggling harder and by self-denigration. That is when we, like Pema, benefit from taking a fresh look at our circumstance and ourselves. As we do, we just may discover by acknowledging our courage to face the immediate obstacle, we, too, have succeeded, not failed. And, as we allow ourselves to bask in the warmth of our sense of success, the obstacle we face, like Pema's persistent, deep anxiety, may disappear. Our final success, it seems, is more a matter of how we view ourselves and others than anything else.

Quite some time ago, as a much younger person, I severely disappointed myself because I arrogantly retreated from guests at a gathering hosted by friends of an aunt and uncle I was visiting in Cuernavaca, Mexico, during the Christmas season of 1980. The guests, retirees all, seemed eager to meet and chat with me, but I did not want to spend time with them. They were, I thought, emotionally needy and physically unappealing. Later that night, alone and ruing such atypical behavior for me, I wrote the following and have lived its meaning ever since (Silverman, 1979):

You and I

The dead, the dying
The sick, the lame
The troubled, the hopeless
The joyless, the insane.

They are our other selves.
They are you and I.
Touch them and they vanish.
Kiss them and they die.

There is a frequently told story about a legendary Tibetan Buddhist meditation master and teacher, Milarepa, who had been called upon by local residents in an area of Tibet haunted by ghosts and spirits to rid the area of an especially fierce spirit which frightened and possessed many of the people. Earlier, they had asked several teachers to dispel the spirit. All used incantations, prayers, and other mystical methods, but none had been successful. Milarepa undaunted by the apparent difficulty of the challenge went to encounter the troublesome spirit. In short order, he returned to report that the spirit would no longer bother them. Grateful, yet incredulous, they asked, *"How did you send it away?"* He quietly replied, *"I didn't. It's still there. I spoke to it and learned it wanted a friend. So I became its friend."* By showing kindness and respect to the spirit through thoughtful listening and by offering compassionate care, he helped transform its fierce and fearsome aspects into something quite benign, accomplishing what others who had chosen to struggle with it had not..

Tsultrim Allione (2008) captured and modernized this idea of acceptance and has honed it as a method for dispelling our own inner demons, not just those we encounter outside ourselves. She outlines how and when to apply kindness to these fearsome demons we learn to visualize and with whom we learn to communicate to incorporate them into our being rather than hiding from them or pushing them away. When we learn to accept them as allies in disguise, we are apt to find the peace and contentment we seek.

Kindness Differs from Indulgence. Essentially kindness, as applied to personal change, refers to unconditional acceptance. We see what we have done, the good, the bad, and the ugly and accept it all, thinking, *"OK. It's OK. It's all right."* This is a little like the transactional analysis (Harris, 2004) approach to personal growth. Not that we condone thought-behavior links that harm ourselves or others. We do not. We choose to accept them as signs of how we functioned *at a particular time*, data we can examine to lead us to the personal changes most helpful and apt for us to launch. As such, we welcome such knowledge as a teacher guiding us toward a more satisfying life, nothing more, nothing less. If, on the other hand, if we reject rather than accept what we consider as undesirable aspects of ourselves, we shrivel rather than enlarge and solidify rather than flow. As we may come to believe we can not behave differently than we have, we settle and suffer endlessly. Acceptance of ourselves "warts and all" is at the core of being kind to ourselves and propels and supports our continuing growth.

Indulgence, on the other hand, momentarily satisfies our desire to escape from or avoid our awareness of what we consider undesirable about ourselves. Indulgence helps keep us stuck by assuaging our angry, hurt, or fearful feelings instead of resolving them. We indulge ourselves when we tunnel through a half-gallon carton of chocolate fudge frozen yogurt spoonful-by-spoonful even after we no longer can taste its chocolate coolness; down mug-after-mug of beer with friends during a club night until we vomit all over ourselves; and buy clothing and accessories we do not need nor can we afford. Indulgence of this sort brings fleeting comfort while occasioning longer-lasting discomfort that comes from weight-gain, physical pain and discomfort, and self-loathing. Accepting ourselves, no matter what we have done, then choosing to move on along a surer path to happiness is the greatest kindness we can show ourselves.

The fruits of kindness are contentment and spaciousness. The fruits of indulgence are unhappiness and constriction.

Compassion Differs from Sympathy. Some enter personal service fields, such as nursing, social work, and speech-language pathology, driven by feelings of pity for those whose daily life resembles a struggle for recognition and accomplishment. I was one of those individuals. Still harboring hurt and resentment over legions of trials I faced from the age of three on, I vowed to prevent others, especially children, from facing similar ones. My goal: Remove their pain, the pain of exclusion, the pain of isolation, and the pain of hurt that ineffective speech skills can bring. Working at stripping away the pain that I thought was theirs consumed me. Eventually, I recognized that dealing with my own related pain provided the strength and insight needed to help them deal with their own pain in their own way.

Compassion leads to skilled action based on clear understanding that liberates; whereas sympathy, often based on projection, imprisons. Offering compassion communicates belief in the capacity to learn and grow unlike the offering of sympathy, or pity, that generally conveys a certain hopelessness (e.g., Silverman, 2006b).

How long it may take to achieve our final goals can not be known when we start out, but, once we start, we should keep on (e.g., Gimian, 2008). Changing as we wish may take weeks; it may take months; it may take years; it may take decades. What we do know is that it will not be a smooth journey, especially when older beliefs and behaviors resurface in circumstances where they are stronger than desirable, newly-emerging ones. At those times, we may believe the change we have worked so hard to accomplish may not be possible. But that is not necessarily true. Such times only tell us we need to stick to our commitment because we may not yet have done all we can. That is all. There is no need for anger, or blame, or sadness. We are simply human, as the late composer Jerome Kern and the late lyricist Dorothy Fields remind us in their classic song, "Pick Yourself Up," by advising us when we have fallen to, "*. . . Pick yourself up, dust yourself off, then start all over again. . .*" Or, as Hasidic Jews say, "*The tzadik (righteous person) falls seven times and rises seven times.*"

Like those who find it helpful to reinforce their commitment to a long and arduous trek by periodically stopping to look back to see and appreciate how far they already have traveled, we, too, can benefit from pausing occasionally, especially when we think we are failing, to notice and acknowledge our already indisputable successes. Then, like the long-haul trekkers we may be, we recommence our journey placing one foot in front of the other again and again until we reach our destination. Hard as it may be on occasion, persevering, we arrive!

PART II

BELIEFS THAT FACILLITATE DESIRED CHANGE

The following five chapters each present beliefs that facilitate desired personal change. When internalized, each helps establish greater self-respect, tolerance, and harmony, without which the management of desired change rarely succeeds. There are other beliefs which contribute to these identical outcomes, but, in my opinion, these are key. If, in your work, you do not already value Partnering clients and caregivers over Rescuing them, experience the reality of self-sufficiency, strive for empathetic understanding and compassionate care, appreciate the relativity of the concepts, "right" and "wrong," and seek to fashion new behavior from current strengths, a strategy to which all the other beliefs in these chapters point, perhaps, they will encourage you to do so. And please note: Chapters 3 through 6 individually provide specific direction for implementing Partnering, discussed in Chapter 2, as an orientation of choice for providing satisfying clinical service.

2   RESCUING, NO. PARTNERING, YES.

Of the beliefs I cultivated to shape my approach to clinical work, the first, because it is so elemental, was: *Rescuing[1] interferes with growth. Partnering[2] enhances it.* This awareness arose from my experience as a Transactional Analysis (TA) trainee. Within the TA framework, interacting with clients as Rescuer was soundly discouraged because such interaction severely limits, if not obliterates, clients' personal power. Stemming, as it does, from the therapist's belief, *"I, not the client, know what is best for the client."* Rescuing rarely leads to change the client desires. What it fashions is an unhealthy, co-dependent clinical relationship. With that awareness guiding me, I reconstructed my perception of an effective clinical role as a speech-language pathologist from that of Rescuer, which I recognized I had assumed from Day 1, to that of Partner.

The Pitfalls of Rescuing

You may be wondering, *"What is so bad about rescuing?'* since, in everyday society, we consider rescuing to be admirable, even heroic. We are grateful to firemen for removing trapped or immobile people from burning buildings; lifeguards for pulling cramping swimmers from lakes; paramedics for saving people experiencing cardiac arrhythmia; and ordinary citizens for performing heroic acts of selflessness, such as foiling a mugging, returning lost wallets intact, or alerting neighbors to an early morning fire in their apartment building. But would we consider firemen who set fire to peoples' homes so they could rescue them or who pulled people from burning office buildings only to toss them back in so they could rescue them again and again helpful? Obviously, not. We would consider them, at the very least, to be menaces. These outlandish examples of pseudo-rescuers relating to others as props to satisfy their own needs actually resemble Rescuers in real-life who find ways to serve primarily to satisfy their own needs to feel worthwhile. You may know some by stereotype, e.g., *The Helicopter Parent*, *The Martyr*, and *The Enabler*. People exemplifying these archetypes are not necessarily malevolent. In fact, they could be you. They were me. Rescuers are people who really want to help. What Rescuers need to learn is how best to do that for the welfare of others and for their own sakes. And they can.

Rescuing as an Unproductive Lifestyle. Rescuers adopt Rescuing as a lifestyle (Berne, 1996) to meet their subconscious needs. Giving elaborate gifts they cannot afford when simple ones would not only be accepted but desirable; offering unsolicited, unnecessary monetary gifts to family and friends that bring discomfort and embarrassment to the recipients; and voluntarily performing tasks others neither request nor desire, such as raking leaves from a neighbor's lawn or trimming a neighbor's hedge, reinforce a sense of self-importance and indispensability with the possible intent of manipulating the recipients of their intrusive actions into offering them goods, services, and, even, friendship. Rescuing can be quite subtle yet lethal. For instance, someone I know almost always greets me by asking, *"How are you feeling?"* She asks this somewhat common-place question in a quiet, soothing voice combined with a penetrating glance to convey deep concern. The effect of her words, voice, and manner are always unsettling for me conveying, as they do, that she knows something troubling me I need to share with her so she can help me, something of which I may be unaware, but, because of her keen desire to be helpful to me, something she already has detected by invading my private space. This calculated approach to convince me to open up to her encourages both self-doubt and fear implying she knows me better than I know myself. So, when she asks how I am feeling, I deflect her trolling through my psyche for personal information with a terse, *"Fine. How are you?"* I have learned that to admit to her I am feeling sub-par or facing a challenge at work or in a personal relationship leads me to feel sorry for myself, and then my mood and energy plummet. But she persists. She repeats almost soulfully, *"How are you feeling --- REALLY?"* I hold firm, defending myself from her prying because I recognize she needs to appear to want to offer help to feel strong. To feel strong, she needs to encourage me to feel weak. As I insist I am feeling fine, she quickly exits. Game over, temporarily.

We need to consider the effect we have on clients and caregivers when we begin a meeting by asking, *"How are you feeling?"* We, too, may be subconsciously placing ourselves in the role of Rescuer so we can feel strong. We, too, may be inadvertently weakening another by implying we know them better than they know themselves, and they need us to be all right whereas a Partner encourages clients to acknowledge that they are all right even if they temporarily need our help to be the best they can be.

Often Rescuers, as do most of us, relate to others as projections of ourselves (Please see the section, "Projections," in Chapter 1). Rescuers attempt to provide the relief for others they wish they had for themselves. This can be an upside of Rescuing. For instance, in January, 2007, Oprah Winfrey opened a school in South Africa for 152 young girls residing there to train them for leadership positions. She specifically constructed the school to be beautiful because she believes beauty inspires. A goal was for these girls to experience what she had not as a girl. On a less grand scale, the first year I worked as a speech therapist I became re-united with an aunt to whom I had been exceptionally close as an infant and toddler. My aunt, a very perceptive person, awakened my self-awareness by telling me, after carefully listening to me passionately describe my work with autistic preschoolers, *"You are helping them to help yourself. You know their pain."* She knew I had stuttered severely as a young child and been made to live and feel like an outsider after the death of my mother, her sister. She knew no one had helped me speak, grieve the loss of my mother, or feel like a cherished member of my nuclear family. Many who decide early in life or later on to be of service do so to prevent or reduce for others pain they personally have known.

This is common knowledge. It is the source of inventions, innovations, legislation, and social, economic, and political revolutions. But the downside of such Rescuing can be that subconsciously, like me, Rescuers reinforce their belief they have no right to have needs of their own or to have them met directly. We use others as stand-in's. In that way, Rescuers neither genuinely help those they purport to aid nor find the deep relief they seek from ministering to others. And, instead of finding satisfaction, they frequently face rejection from those whose independence they stymied rather than nurtured when those individuals develop the awareness of having been squelched and the ability to rebel. Think of those you know who, rather than relating warmly and with kindness to dictatorial parents, suffocating partners, and domineering employers, do what they feel they need to do to escape such alleged oppressors, often without a backward look. The payoff for Rescuers is bitterness and for those they manipulate, distrust of others

Not all clients, caregivers, colleagues, and others appreciated working with me as a Partner, especially those whose personal agendas directed them to seek out a Rescuer. But I persevered. I entered into treatment agreements primarily with those who sought a collaborative environment within which to create personal change. I discovered quite soon that, as a Partner, I more easily facilitated change for clients and caregivers and maintained my own health.

Hopefully, this chapter will help you make the same discovery, or, at least, lead you to a deeper understanding of the ramifications that choosing a clinical role has on professional accountability and job satisfaction and longevity.

RESCUING AS DISTINCT FROM PARTNERING

Like other clinicians, I sometime encounter requests from working clinicians wanting help solving current clinical dilemmas. The following illumines key elements of Partnering as distinguished from Rescuing:

> *I am currently treating a client who is 39 years old and has never before received speech therapy for her stuttering problem. We have had three sessions, and I see her as lacking motivation. She has not completed homework. It appears she expects me to "fix" the problem. What can help motivate her and help her to realize her role and responsibility?*

In response, I frequently advise a change in therapist outlook and orientation. For example, here is the kind of message I am prone to send someone with that stated need:

Our focus can be primarily on fixing clients' problems or addressing their needs. While, superficially, the approaches may seem one and the same, they are not. From my knowledge and experience, unless a client, child or adult feels known by the therapist and fully engaged in the therapy process, their commitment is insufficient to establish the change they want. In those circumstances where clients feel like foot soldiers working for therapists functioning as Commanding Generals seeking victory over The Problem, the clients often go AWOL one way or another, i.e., through poor attendance, non-compliance, and/or flaming e-mails announcing departures from the program.

So, the therapist's job is first and foremost to connect with the client to establish a teammate, together with whom, and only together with whom, meaningful change can be identified and achieved.

Although the clinician requested help fixing the client, in my view, it was the clinician who first needed to change because the client is seemingly rejecting her manner of service. Choosing whether we believe our work is to fix problems or help people help themselves is *the* decision we all make as therapists, consciously or subconsciously. All others flow from that perspective, including whether and when to begin treatment; treatment goals; methods to apply; the frequency of treatments; whether individual, group, or a combination of the two treatment-types best advances treatment goals; the estimated length of the treatment program; the role of caregivers and other intimates; and so forth. If we believe we are to be a fixer of peoples' problems, we probably see our role as that of *Rescuing* (Berne, 1996). If we believe we are to be a helper to people with problems, we probably see our role as that of *Partnering*. The two seemingly similar beliefs create quite different outcomes.

In a simple, yet riveting, manner, the movie *The Kid* (2000) entertainingly distinguishes Rescuing from Partnering.

Through the magic of the moon and the urgency of his own personal discontent, accentuated by the imminent arrival of his 40th birthday, Russ, the main character, a successful image consultant, unexpectedly encounters Rusty, his despised chubby, awkward, fearful, self-deprecating, lateral lisping, eight-year-old self. Russ trim, smartly dressed, and tyrannical decides he must mold this personally repulsive child into one he can accept for his alter ego to experience the happy childhood he did not.

He restricts what Rusty eats and heavily criticizes his thinking and behavior. Already unhappy because of his beleaguered, friendless school life and harsh rejection from his father, Rusty unblinkingly notes the lonely, joyless adult life awaiting him, the antithesis of what he wishes to have and be, and becomes increasingly distressed. Yet he maintains a strained communication with Russ, partly to try to reform *him* into being the adult he wants to be.

Neither succeeds in their attempt to fix the other part of themselves. Each, hurt and angry, increasingly retreats sullenly into himself until Russ mobilizes himself to seek a solution to this unwelcome disturbance in his otherwise sterile life by consulting with an acquaintance. Taking her advice, he ceases trying to mold Rusty into an acceptable version of his eight-year-old self and begins collaborating with him as he is. As Russ becomes an ally to help him find his way back to the time-space co-ordinate he left, Rusty enthusiastically shares essential personal information. Their mutual respect for each other as collaborators, depicted as increasing warmth and friendliness to each other, heightens their individual feelings of self-worth. Together they find the way home for a newly strong, confident Rusty and a long-desired adventure for the renewed, self-accepting Russ.

When Russ and Rusty tried to Rescue each other, they resisted one another. They pushed each other away. Neither got what he wanted as he became more entrenched in self-righteousness, self-pity, and self-centeredness. When they Partnered with each other, they came together to resolve a critical need. Although Russ did not expect or realize their collaboration would benefit him personally, he became more open, kind, joyful, and self-accepting as he unselfishly practiced genuine altruism. That helped him find the way to a life for which he had longed.

We know that to do our job well we need to conceptualize our role as that of Partner, but the tendency for us individually and collectively to subconsciously believe we provide actual help rather than short-term relief by acting as Rescuer is so strong that Lao Tzu, the founder of Taoism who lived in the 4th Century B.C., constructed the following proverb to help re-direct that empathetic knee-jerk impulse to help as Rescuer to help as Partner,

"Give a man a fish, and you have fed him for today.

Teach a man to fish, and you have fed him for a lifetime."

Rescuing almost always hurts those involved. Partnering almost always helps them grow into the fullness of their being.

RESCUING AS IT IS

Invitations to Rescue

Occasionally, we rescue. We buy a steaming cup of hot chocolate for a Salvation Army bell-ringer shifting his body weight from leg-to-leg to avoid freezing on a blustery December day. We clear our elderly neighbor's driveway of snow after a crippling blizzard. Or we offer to stay with a neighbor's sick child so the parent can go to work. We make these gestures selflessly or, possibly, with an expectation of a spiritual reward, such as down-payment on a star in our Crown in Heaven or to increase our accumulation of *mitzvah*-points. But, in either case, we do so matter-of-factly with awareness, then move on. We recognize and imply this is a one-time gesture we were pleased to make and that we harbor no expectations for, nor are we seeking, a relationship based on need.

As a therapist, we need to be especially wary of making such choices too quickly without awareness because a seemingly ordinary circumstance or request can function as an *Invitation to Rescue*. Some requests, tacit or expressed, possess the capability of hooking us through our unrecognized vulnerabilities into co-creating a dependency relationship, and, unless we understand our motivations for proceeding, we may find ourselves taking the bait and unhappily hooked. For instance, consider the following two e-mail's I received from strangers in just the past two weeks. I edited each to help preserve the writers' privacy. To me, one was a patent Invitation to Rescue while the other was an ordinary request for assistance. Which do you think was which?

E-mail Number 1- From A Parent

Dear Ellen-Marie,

I read your profile on the People Page of the ASHA Leader, and I am so inspired. I am a speech pathologist who has a son diagnosed with Selective Mutism. Arthur is six years old and attends first grade in our local public elementary school. Although he has done remarkably well (will now freely speak in school to his teacher, is extremely verbose in the 'speech room,' and will talk to peers when prompted), he continues to have an extremely difficult time in other social settings. Birthday parties and doctors' appointments are disastrous! The social anxiety literally paralyzes him, and he has started to exhibit some immature behaviors (crawling behind the curtains or standing on the coffee table) if he feels "uncomfortable." He also has quite a significant articulation delay, of which he has become very aware of and protective of himself if he thinks someone will not understand him. I practice speech (and we live) in the suburbs of Abbotville. I was wondering if you have any resources or suggestions to offer

Thanks,

Amelé S.

And

E-mail Number 2 – From An Adult with a Stuttering Problem

Hi Ellen-Marie,

I am a covert stutterer of 27, and I don't want to go into describing what stuttering has done to me. If not for the fact that I am a Christian and understand what committing suicide entails, I don't think . . . .

I just read your article of 2003, sorry but I almost stopped reading after the first two paragraphs where you said you didn't realize you were a stutterer 'til the age of 37. At first I thought 'this person doesn't know what it truly means to be a stutterer otherwise how could she not have known.'

I was merely comparing you to myself as I think I have stuttered since I was five and have felt the pain all the way knowing full well that I am a stutterer. I apologize for the prejudice; your case might be rare but I appreciate that no two stutterers are the same. I continued to read through your article due to my interest in meditation and found that you really have something to offer.

I had earlier started the simple form of meditation- just observing and welcoming my thoughts for at least 30 minutes a day. I found it hard to follow through so I stopped and tried out some other method. Honestly, I think that is part of my problems; all my life I have been trying out new things in the hope of finding a solution to my stuttering. I have never persevered with one method for more than three weeks. However, I think I can recall that while I was practicing the meditation, I felt a lot better as a person. Now I am willing to go back and commit to it.

The reason I am writing is to ask for your help in providing a source of information by which I can practice meditation with the aim of becoming a better person and resolving my stutter. I am at that state in my life (with a Master's Degree) where I have to make career decisions but feel so constrained to do anything because I am a stutterer. It is painful, really painful. Please help me.

Looking forward to hearing from you,

Daniel

If you thought I thought E-Mail number 2 was the invitation, we agree.

E-mail Number 1 is a fairly typical request for more personalized information. I sometimes receive these after I make a presentation to a group or publish an article. In this case, the writer implies she will be doing what she thinks needs to be done and hopes that may be enhanced by an additional tidbit of information from me.

E-mail Number 2, on the other hand, screams, *"Watch Out!"* primarily because of the reference to suicide in the second sentence. I have learned that such an early, unsolicited emotionally gripping disclosure by a stranger can be a serious gambit to Rescue by tempting the therapist to assume responsibility not only for another's well-being but very existence. A would-be client with such a motivation frequently is less inclined to work for personal change than in hurting, shaming, and embarrassing the therapist enticed to help. A wish is to graphically and painfully demonstrate, especially to the therapist, their inadequate knowledge and skill. Behind this wish is the desire to experience a power-over success with a therapist as compensation for a succession of previous, dissatisfying therapy experiences that left them feeling disempowered.

Other suggestions that Daniel was offering an Invitation to Rescue, rather than genuinely seeking assistance changing are:

1) The statement *". . . you really have something to offer."* --- suggesting

    I can be *the* one to help him, i.e., flattery;

2) The reference to never having been able to commit for more than

    "three weeks" to a program of change --- a challenge

    to prove myself better than his previous therapists, i.e., enticement;

3) The emphatic declaration he is living in considerable *"pain"* because

    stuttering prevents him from making necessary life choices

    to feel content --- explicit avowal of himself as Victim,[3] i.e., invitation; and

4) The final, direct request and invitation, *"Please help me."* in case

    I somehow missed the meaning of the e-mail, concluding with,

    "Look forward to hearing from you." i.e., an avowal of dependence

    on me to put things right for him.

Daniel either was desperate for assistance or desperately wanted me to believe he was and that I was *the* one to provide it. He presents himself as Victim depending on a Rescuer to make his life better rather than assistance to do that for himself. An alternative approach to soliciting help, such as Amelé's above, that bodes well for the possibility of a favorable speech therapy partnership, is one that includes a straight-forward request for guidance to help achieve "x," "y," and/or "z."

Now, please do not think of me as cynical and uncaring. I do care about Daniel and those like him who seem willing to sacrifice long-term personal well-being for a contrived short-lived feeling of superiority over someone they lure into service as a helper or guide. But I have learned only to offer what I think may be of real help rather than attempting to satisfy expressed requests at face value. This is the reply I e-mailed him:

> *Hello, Daniel,*
>
> *You sound like a very intelligent person, Daniel, who is well-read in general and in the area of stuttering. My suggestion to you at this time would be to talk about your concerns, your pain, your anxieties making personal choices with someone faith-based. Such an individual also may be able to help you begin and maintain a Christian-based mediation practice, such as centering prayer.*
>
> *Best wishes.*

I hope Daniel finds the help he needs and that I may have steered him in a useful direction by side-stepping what I considered to be his *Invitation to Rescue* to refer him to the kind of professional with the discernment and other requisite skills likely to help him grow. Recall: He opened his request by declaring he is a Christian. And, please note: Whenever someone states or implies that they are considering suicide, it is essential to take their avowal seriously and to make a prompt referral to a professional trained in addressing such a circumstance. In this situation, a clergy person seemed the most appropriate source of help.

The nature of Daniel's appeal for help unfortunately is not rare among adults seeking therapy to address their stuttering problems, except for the overt suicidal reference. Adults with stuttering problems, who first experience therapy as a child yet continue to wrestle with the problem as an adult, frequently are quite angry. A significant amount of their anger derives from feeling betrayed by speech therapy and the therapists who implicitly promised help but did not deliver. Some stems from feeling personally responsible for their lack of or limited personal change leading them to the mistakenly conclude they are hopeless and helpless, a belief capable of generating much anger and some angst.

The attitude of many adults with stuttering problems toward speech therapy directs us to carefully consider how we wish to portray ourselves as professionals. Reflecting on the short- and long-range impact the role of therapist can have on us, our clients, and their caregivers, can lead us to eschew imaging ourselves as Rescuer and conceptualize our functioning as that of Partner since evidence convincingly shows that people change themselves. Professionals can only responsibly point the way.

The dynamics of therapist-child relationships can easily foster the relative powerlessness of a child in relation to an adult, thereby, grooming the child to act as Victim. But this is not a necessary element of treatment as seen in *Jason's Secret* (Silverman, 2001), the novel I authored for children and caring adults. The novel details 10 year-old Jason Loring's efforts to hide his stuttering and his relationship with the school speech therapist. In Chapter 9, I portray exchanges between the therapist and Jason in which she cast Jason as a Partner in the enterprise with whom details of therapy were negotiated. The following is an excerpt from the chapter when Jason reluctantly meets the therapist in her office for the first time (Silverman, 2001, pp. 97-100).

'. . . I don't want speech therapy,' Jason exclaimed. 'Everyone will think I'm stupid.'

'Jason, no one thinks you're stupid. But it doesn't matter what they think. What you think matters. You know you're not stupid,' she repeated looking at him hard.

'Yeh-yeah,' Jason acknowledged. He didn't think he was stupid.

He knew he was pretty smart. But he couldn't understand why he stuttered and couldn't stop. That made him feel stupid. He didn't know why everyone else could talk right, but he couldn't. He couldn't figure that out.

'So you have to do the right thing. You need help. You need to accept it,' she added. I couldn't stop (stuttering) until a speech therapist showed me how.'

'I-I-I-I weh-went to a speech therapist in the first grade. It didn't help.'

'Oh? . . . '

'She made me talk 'turtle talk.' I hated that. It made me feel stupid.'

'Well, we won't do that now. Times are different. By the way,' she smiled. 'I don't talk like a turtle. Do I?'

'NNNnnno!'

Jason sunk into the recliner and drew in a long breath. She didn't talk like a turtle. She talked normal. And she had a good voice.

'Well, you-you don't have to talk like a turtle either,' she continued. I'll teach you about talking and show you how to talk smoothly. You'll have to practice a lot though. What do you say?'

Jason wasn't sure what to say. He wanted to stop stuttering. That was sure. Maybe her way would work. But he didn't want people to think he was a freak because he went to speech therapy. 'I doh-don't . . . '

'You don't . . . ?'

' . . . I don't know. I guess so,' he said. He really wanted to talk like everyone else. And he was beginning to like Dr. Allen. He'd deal with that freak thing later if he had to.

'Good decision, Jason. We need to find a time to meet here three times each week,' she smiled. 'What class don't you mind missing for a while?'

Jason thought hard. He thought he might not mind missing math.

But he liked it. Then he thought missing writing class would be better until he thought about making up the assignments. That could be hard. He couldn't decide. Suddenly he had an idea. 'How-how about before school? I can get here early . . . '

'I have meetings then,' she replied scanning her calendar. 'How about right before lunch?'

That was math. He didn't want to miss it. 'Uh-how about after school?'

'Let's try this,' Dr. Allen suggested. 'This month we'll meet before home room on Monday's and Wednesday's and before lunch on Friday's.

That will get us started. I'll change some of my early morning appointments,' she said writing in her calendar.

'Fruh-Friday's before lunch is math.' Jason added. 'I doh-don't want to miss that.'

'Who's your math teacher?'

'Muh-Mrs. Kingsley.'

'I'll talk to her about our meeting plans. I'm sure she'll help you make up Friday math classes. Okay?'

'Oh-okay,' he said.

This type of negotiation where client and therapist make mutually agreeable decisions about working together reflects the therapist's belief that clients are Partners not recipients of therapy. Within that framework, they are free to be. They do not dance the Rescue Dance.

The Rescue Dance

This dance involves three steps: Coming together, Changing roles, and Angrily Breaking apart as illustrated in the following scenario excerpted from Silverman (2001c):

> Steve, a 29 year-old, who has enrolled in therapy almost continually since he was six when he began stuttering reading aloud in class, feels the need to resume treatment. Despite the fact he is successful in a responsible position, has a partner in life, and enjoys a cordial circle of friends, he feels he could be more successful if he no longer stuttered.
>
> He places himself in the role of Victim searching for a therapist (Rescuer) by verbally and non-verbally saying to those he contacts, 'I need your help. Only you can help me be happy.' But Steve, in so doing, is not honest with himself. He really believes no one 'out there' is able to change him from a person who stutters into someone who does not. In fact, Steve believes that since no speech therapist has cured him, none ever will. And the experience he really wants is to enjoy shaming and humiliating any therapist who takes his Victim bait to try. He accomplishes that by entering a therapy relationship then skillfully resisting almost all the suggestions and recommendations the therapist makes, until frustrated by her inability to engage and change him she dismisses him. That is when he directly notifies her he has not benefited from treatment and has wasted his time and money. The dance ends leaving the therapist angry and, possibly, hurt because she feels her efforts were misunderstood and rejected. She feels like a failure distressed enough to consider refusing treatment to adults who have stuttering problems. She changed roles from Rescuer to Victim. And Steve, feeling superior as the game ends because he has scored the telling wound, feels triumphant at having shown the therapist know just how incompetent he thinks she is. He changed roles from Victim to Persecutor.[4] But, after a short while, he resumes feeling his usual sadness when he once again entertains his belief that he is incurable.

The empathetic therapist, recognizing and identifying with Steve's pain, seeks to relieve it to help him and to feel better, too. But failing to distinguish between her own perception of his pain and his actual pain, she probably does not provide him with the help he actually needs (Silverman, 2006b). Steve may have recognized her difficulty relating to him as a unique individual and selected her as his therapist for just that reason.[5] So, for a while, the two find satisfaction working together, she telling and showing him what he needs to do to change and he listening attentively to what she says. But this pleasant interval is short-lived. When Steve can no longer contain his actual motivation for engaging in treatment with her, he reverts to his true face, that of revenge-seeker, to sabotage her efforts to Rescue him. Their almost idyllic fantasy relationship erupts into painful disarray, similar to a Moliere farce, as Victim becomes Persecutor and Rescuer becomes Victim.

Steve was correct: *No one "out there" can change him.* That is his job. But, until he believes that is true and lives that belief, after learning that is simply the way it is, he will continue to suffer, and so will the therapists who try to change him. Eventually, we learn that clients can learn to meet their own needs and that teaching them to do that is our job. That is when we embrace the role of Partner and become truly helpful and personally satisfied (Zukav, 1999).

PARTNERING AS IT IS

In the "Special Features" section on the DVD of the comedic whodunit film *Gosford Park* (2001), several cast and crew members, including the director, Robert Altman, make statements about his unique style, which has been described as improvisational, even though, as the late Mr. Altman stressed, the primary actors' lines in each scene were scripted. The improvisational element involves the key actors freely placing themselves in their scenes then moving appropriately for their characters as the hand-held cameras shift position to seemingly eaves-drop. Mr. Altman believed the actors knew more about the motivations of the characters they portrayed than he did, so he encouraged them to be the characters, not just play them. The actors participating in this post-production forum stated they found this particular collaboration extremely satisfying. Some said Mr. Altman was on most actors' short list of directors with whom they wished to work.

Steven Spielberg also has been described as a director who collaborates with actors. During the December, 2006, televised showing of the Kennedy Center Honors, actor Tom Hanks described honoree, Mr. Spielberg, as having shared his own fears and vulnerabilities with him during the filming of *Saving Private Ryan* (1998). Mr. Hanks remarked that Mr. Spielberg's admission had been liberating for him.

Our role resembles that of a film director. Like directors, we, too, develop stories (Silverman, 2004), people's life stories. We help them remove obstacles and learn skills to freely live their lives' dreams. While the stories movie directors tell become seemingly frozen in time, the stories we tell continue to evolve far beyond our active involvement encouraging their unfoldment. And, like, films clients' stories may be inspiring or horrifying, or both. They may be comedic. They may seem Gothic or like science fiction. They may involve dawning self-awareness and redemption or terminal naiveté. They may be developed into sequels. But they always result from a team effort where we, like film directors, oversee the contributions of those involved, as few as two or as many as 10 or more. If we wish to help create the body of quality work that academy award winning directors Robert Altman and Steven Spielberg have, then we, too, may wish to deliberately work as they, i.e., collaborator with our teams.

Partnering allows and encourages others to be their best selves. For instance, men and women in partnership with one another strengthen their relationship when they come to recognize that each gender processes and uses language differently (e.g., Tannen, 2001). Rather than demand that their partner speak as they do, wise men and women choose to learn to understand the linguistic and metalinguistic forms their partners use to present their ideas and feelings. Similarly, we relate to members of different cultural, social, and religious groups by acknowledging, embracing, and accepting our mutual differences and similarities. Partners provide information and direction to each other but stop short of imposing their standards on another because they believe that is unwise. Consider the following speech therapy experience of the wife of a colleague of mine.

> *In 1973, I was hired as an assistant professor of communication disorders in the School of Speech at a Midwestern university. An assistant professor in the interpersonal communications program of that School, hired the same year, frequently needled me during School meetings about the practice of school-based speech therapists. Jim found troubling the then, long-time practice of unilaterally enrolling school children in therapy who failed speech and language screenings and subsequent follow-up testing. He believed enrolling children in therapy because they lisped, then re-enrolling them semester after semester when they failed to speak without lisping was more damaging than if they had not been entered into speech therapy in the first place. He told me a therapist following this policy had placed his wife in speech therapy when she was a second-grader because she lisped. He believed that practice compromised his wife's self-esteem for quite a long time after that. She told him that before she entered therapy, she thought she was no better or no worse than others. But, when the therapist enrolled her in therapy to speak without lisping, she felt inferior. When discharged several semesters later as no longer improving yet still lisping, she felt ashamed, angry, and embarrassed. She felt ashamed for lisping and failing to learn to stop. She felt angry at herself for not being able to speak like her classmates. And she felt embarrassed to speak in almost all circumstances because she felt inferior to those who did not lisp, which was practically everyone else.*

Practices currently in place to encourage therapists to partner with caregivers and colleagues to jointly reach decisions concerning children's enrollment in school speech therapy programs sharply reduce the possibility more children will experience that kind of emotional damage, at least on a large scale. For the record: I did not defend my unknown colleague to Jim. I expressed my sincere sadness that his wife, as a child, had come to view herself as damaged goods instead of the person of light and charity I had come to know because of the ill-considered actions stemming from an apparently mindless decision by one speech therapist who seemed to consider herself a Rescuer.

The Three P's That Increase Therapist Effectiveness

The three qualities that increase therapist effectiveness, according to Eric Berne (1996), founder of Transactional Analysis and pioneer in the practice of therapist Partnering are: *Potency, Protection, and Permission.* He believed therapists need to be strong, to create environments where their clients feel safe, and to encourage clients to do what they believe is necessary for their own sakes.

Potency. Appearing powerful may seem a contradictory posture for a therapist committed to Partnering to cultivate. Such a wish may seem characteristic of one who wishes to rule. But equate potency with self-confidence, decisiveness, and knowledge to appreciate the desirable qualities implied. Who would want to work with a therapist who appeared confused and uncertain about their role and uninformed about key matters relevant to desired personal change? Very few, except possibly those who, for personal reasons, choose to engage in a relationship with a student-in-training. But, even then, these clients know a qualified professional supervises the student. So, they place their confidence in the university or college training program based on its merits, not the student.

Trust contributes mightily to therapy success. And it needs to be earned. Sigmund Freud, for example, reportedly stressed that the wise therapist refrains from expecting trust at the outset, which, he cautions, can create a burden for the client. He offered that trust well-placed evolves from relating to the therapist over time while trusting in advance portends psychosis (Ahlskog, 2001). While external accoutrements such as office location, office furnishings, university affiliations, the title "doctor" or "professor," and charging higher fees than competitors may imply quality, faith that the therapist possesses the ability to be helpful derives more readily from interacting with a confident, knowledgeable professional than one who relies primarily on props to convey that impression. And, though it may seem contradictory, cultivating meekness, not weakness, contributes to creating a climate of trust because it resonates genuine personal strength. When therapists place client and caregivers foremost in the interchange rather than highlighting their own sublime qualities, they focus clients and caregivers on meeting their own needs rather distracting them from that critical work by, perhaps, unwittingly encouraging an unproductive interest in themselves.

Brett Favre, the legendary quarterback and anticipated football Hall-of-Fame honoree, joined the New York Jets in 2008 following their disappointing 2007 season when they won four games but lost twelve. The confidence in himself and in the team he exudes has inspired his new teammates. A starting member of the offense reportedly said, *"Looking into his eyes in the huddle, I see his confidence and, seeing that, I raise my level of play."* In November of 2008, as I write this, the Jets enjoy newly found respect as first place holders in Eastern Division of the American Football Conference.

During the final hour of my last day as team leader and senior therapist at an outpatient rehabilitation program for adults who had suffered traumatic brain injury, the manager of the agency's work-hardening program, which had prepared several of our patients to return to work, came to my office to say, *"Good-Bye."* She wanted me to know she thought I had done well. *"Your patients trusted you,"* she said. *"They really trusted you."* There was nothing more meaningful she could have said to me about my clinical work, a message I had received many times from patients themselves.   For instance:

On that very same day, a proud, young man, DeAngelo, whose sole income came from monthly social security payments, took public transportation, traveling more than an hour each way on a frigid January afternoon, when he had no treatment scheduled, to hand me a greeting card wishing me well.

Several years before, Tony, 29, hemiplegic and non-verbal several years after a motor vehicle accident, made a striking, but not entirely unexpected admission to me during a Christmas Eve Day session. Tony had worked with the speech therapist I replaced, who had obtained the funding to purchase a portable electronic speech aid for him. He seemed to enjoy using the tool, which for recipients of his messages created a mildly frustrating communication experience because of his poor manual control and spelling. Because I noticed he produced audible laughter and other socially appropriate sounds, such as "hmmm," I suspected he might be able to voice his thoughts and feelings. And that was just what he did that late afternoon. I don't remember the off-hand remark he made in breathy, slightly labored speech, but I remember what he said, when I, excited and moved, thinking I was witnessing a Christmas miracle that would be the gift of gifts to his mother, asked whether he would speak to her that evening. He quickly answered, "No." To my stunned, "Why?" he replied, "It's not normal." I was not then or later able to convince him to consider participating in experimental speech therapy to determine whether he could produce speech more to his expectations. But I was deeply touched that he had revealed to me that one afternoon that he could speak.

And, earlier that year, forty-something James, who had significant short-term memory loss, moderate distractibility, reasoning and problem-solving impairments, and a general disinterest in participating in treatment activities, successfully gave a surprise birthday party for me during a group therapy session. The event included a well-lit carrot cake, which he proudly explained he ordered because he heard I was a vegetarian. Staff, who delivered the cake because he was unable to drive, later asserted that the idea and the planning were his entirely. They merely helped out with transportation matters. They were incredulous witnessing his initiation and determination to create the happening. And, like I, they were greatly moved.

Protection. At a very basic level, we need to care for our clients. That means we need to provide a safe environment. I recall an experience with a co-facilitator of a therapy group of 10 or so adults with traumatic brain injury, many of whom experienced impaired mobility in addition to emotional lability and distractibility. During one of our weekly, one-hour sessions, an alarm sounded signaling the need to promptly evacuate the building. We did not know at the time whether that was a practice drill or a real need, so we decided to leave. Without any discussion at the time between us about how to proceed, the co-facilitator, a psychologist, who used an electric scooter for transportation because of the disabling effects he experienced from arthritis, tore out of the therapy room alone. When the group members and I entered the hallway for the long walk to the nearest exit, I spotted him speeding down the corridor far ahead of us. It took quite some time, and I was quite frightened, but I safely herded all members of the group outdoors where the psychologist already was comfortably waiting. This remains for me a graphic example of how we can behave when we fail to take the responsibility we share for our client's safety.

We do all we can to establish safe physical environments for ourselves and our clients. Selecting a meeting location which offers freedom from intrusion, good air quality, suitable air temperature, proper ventilation, and adequate sanitation; using safe, hygienic products and supplies; and providing skill-appropriate opportunities, adequate directions, and necessary reminders, etc. help assure physical safety. We also take steps to guarantee privacy of therapy participation and content of personal disclosures within the therapy room, during telephone conversations, and *via* e-mail and snail mail. We inform patients-to-be and caregivers concerning our handling of privacy matters at the outset and provide reminders as needed during the course of treatment. Taking these measures exemplifies protection. We all long to feel protected when we are vulnerable, and when we sincerely seek help, we are that. That is why those of us with Rescuer tendencies need to be especially scrupulous concerning our motives and behaviors working with clients and caregivers.

Permission. The third "P," providing permission for clients and caregivers to change almost seems like an oxymoron, but permission from the therapist to change often is necessary. Clients seeking help sometimes seem to be sitting on the cusp. Like Janus, the Roman two-faced god of doorways able to look forward and backward simultaneously, clients sometimes appear frozen. With a longing to inhabit a frustration and pain-free future and doubting they can do what is required to achieve that, enough tension exists to render them inactive. They may skip treatment sessions, neglect required practice, or refuse to reach in other ways. For those who received direct and subliminal messages early and often from powerful others, such as parents, caregivers, teachers, librarians, scout leaders, siblings, bullies, and so forth, that the success they envisioned for themselves was unlikely because they did not deserve it or because they lacked the aptitude, skill, or other resources to achieve it, we can make a huge difference. Sometimes they become hampered by their misunderstanding of the diagnoses we apply that leads them to think only what they cannot do and benefit from a fresh, accurate explanation of what they *can* do.

Twenty-ish Sandra, who suffered traumatic brain injury after the bicycle she was riding was hit from behind by a car, sat in a wheelchair positioned at a 30° angle at mealtime to help compensate for her severe difficulty swallowing liquids and solids. A stubborn, prideful woman with a history of mild mental retardation, she had been transferred to my caseload after her previous speech therapist had been unable to encourage her to participate.

I quickly learned Sandra had come to believe she could not remember anything so trying to learn was useless. When asked to perform a task in therapy or in daycare, she generally refused by responding defiantly and with some regret, "I don't remember anything." The second or third time she offered that excuse to me, I quickly countered with, "Yes, you do! You remember bits and pieces." I reminded her of all that I knew that she remembered, for instance, my appearance, my name, the names of her best friends in daycare, the names of her occupational and physical therapists and her physician. Immediately, her entire body softened, and her facial muscles relaxed. She knew the truth when she heard it. And she knew she did remember "bits and pieces" of her life.

At my encouragement, she printed the simple sentence, "I remember bits and pieces." on a lined piece of paper that I placed at the front of her memory notebook. Building on this revelation, which I often asked her to repeat, she, within the three and one-half years we worked together, learned to eat safely sitting upright and to walk with a hemi-walker. When I resigned from the program, she was being considered for employment at a sheltered workshop.

Then there was Santo, who was thrown from his motorcycle when it collided with a car. Also in his 20's, Santo developed a right hemiplegic following the accident as well as memory and cognitive impairments. When I began working with him, he refused to do any paper and pencil task, explaining since he was right-handed, he could no longer write. Not writing severely compromised his ability to benefit from the memory book that was a universal memory aid for the patients in the adult brain injury rehabilitation program. I advised him that while it was true he may be unable to write with his right hand, he could learn to write with his left, and I expected him to do that. Without any argument, he did, although, from time-to-time, as he was gaining fluency as a left-handed writer, he interrupted an activity to ridicule the quality of his penmanship. At those times, I would respond that all that was needed was for him to practice more. He did. And, as he wrote frequent reminders to himself in his memory notebook, he experienced increased benefits from his rehab experience.

By firmly asserting our belief as credible individuals to patients that they can meet certain, well-targeted goals with conscientious effort and persistence, we help release them to mobilize their resources and move forward. We do this as often as it takes to offset the restrictive messages they carry that, like certain radioactive isotopes, may, otherwise, have very long half-lives.

Contracting as a Structure for Partnering

When we consciously negotiate contracts with clients and caregivers to establish the goals and methods of our mutual clinical enterprise, we cement partnering. We usually begin the process when we first meet to discuss treatment options. By guiding them to clearly state their expectations of what they would consider to be a successful time working with us, we tacitly communicate our expectation that they actively participate in the therapy relationship. This helps clear their mental screens of a common misperception that if unacknowledged may run counter to meeting their therapy goals. That misperception is that *we will fix them.*

Clients often expect us to tell them what to do and then badger them to do it because that is the interchange they experienced with other professionals or caregivers. Unless we directly address this nonsensical presumption up front, we may be faced later with their fierce anger if they believe we have not done our job. To circumvent such unpleasantness and potential litigation and to help avert the possibility clients may exit their relationship with us believing they can not achieve what they want, we state directly whether we believe their stated goals are ones we are prepared to address. If not, we consider what alterations of those goals we can accommodate. If we can establish mutually satisfactory goals, we then jointly consider procedures to meet them, i.e., so-called office requirements, such as attendance and cancellation policies and payment procedures, and clinical requirements, such as inter-session practice, to establish mutual consensus regarding the conduct of therapy. The terms may be re-negotiated as necessary. If we can not reach consensus concerning goals or procedures, now having learned what the individuals expect, we can make suitable recommendations to help them locate appropriate help elsewhere.

An example of a non-negotiation between professional and client in healthcare services is a comedic highlight of the Oscar nominated movie for Best Picture of 2006, *Little Miss Sunshine*.   In the film, a robotic hospital grief liaison counselor meets with Richard whose father Edwin died of a drug overdose moments earlier in the ER.   Edwin had been accompanying the family on a motor trip from New Mexico to California to enter his granddaughter, pre-pubescent Olive, in The Little Miss Sunshine Beauty Pageant.   Coldly, the counselor presents Richard with a sheaf of paperwork to be completed to properly dispose of Edwin's body.   Richard complains that taking time to complete the paperwork would disrupt his family's tightly scheduled travel plans.   He suggests possible alternatives.   Stubbornly, the autocratic counselor sarcastically reiterates her demands.   Unwilling to meet these inflexible requirements, Richard, with the help of his wife, teenage son, brother-in-law, and Olive, steals Edwin's corpse to store in the van so they can meet their travel deadlines, after which, they plan to attend to his burial needs.

The grief liaison counselor had no desire to negotiate.   She shrilly presented a series of demands to Richard in a take-it-or-leave-it manner.   He left.   Similarly, when we only present inflexible rules and expectations to clients and caregivers, we are not negotiating.   We are dictating, and we may be creating parallel opportunities for rebellion.   However, there are occasions when we may have no other choice.   For instance, as employees of hospitals, agencies, school systems, private practices, etc., we rarely have the opportunity to negotiate fees and terms of payment or all desirable treatment options, such as group treatment to supplement individual therapy, off-site based treatment, and so on.   And, if asked by nurses to address the health needs of a nursing home resident with dementia and recently diagnosed aspiration pneumonia and no living will or power of attorney for healthcare, we may choose to unilaterally put our best recommendations into place to address the patient's chewing and swallowing problem.   And so on.

When we can contract to partner, we view the opportunity as if through a wide-angle lens that captures the biggest over-all picture and with a genuine willingness to negotiate. *We do not enter the discussion intent on winning-over potential clients or caregivers to our point-of-view* (Silverman, 2003c).   (Please see Chapters 5 & 6.)   After all, one point-of-view is no better than any other.   If we believe we know the course of action best for a client or caregiver, we are thinking like a Rescuer.   Instead, we listen to clients' and caregivers' needs and expectations, level of commitment and available resources; we express our position; and we each compromise to create workable procedures that can satisfy all participants.   This helps establish the *mutuality* of the enterprise, which, of itself, is a novel and healing experience for those who previously have been encouraged to assume a passive role relating to other helping professionals.   This way we Partner.   We share relevant information.   Then, putting clients' needs first and foremost, we compromise.

Final agreements can be written wholly or in part.   For instance, we can provide each client or caregiver with only a single sheet of paper summarizing payment matters, including attendance and cancellation policies, to be signed and dated or we can present a written summary of all agreements, also to be signed and filed. The value of a complete signed contract increases with time. As clients' and caregivers' memories of the pre-contract discussion fade and enthusiasm to persevere may dim, we can review the document and recall all accomplishments since starting the program to renew motivation. As we examine the contract, we may reconsider goals and methods. Perhaps, when we concluded it, we lacked certain historical information recently made available. Maybe, we need to reconsider the weighting of information available during the time of negotiation. With a mutually agreed upon signed document as a reference point, we are able to make a thoughtful assessment of present and future goals and procedures.

Why contract? We use the tool of contracting to launch and structure our partnering when the overall circumstances permit at least some negotiation. The very process of negotiating helps establish mutuality, or team-building. The contract itself provides a self-regulating tool.

Why negotiate? We use the process of negotiation to empower people to meet their own needs. The process highlights the relevance of identifying our needs, articulating them, and wisely and effectively addressing them with the help of others as needed. So, to do our job as Partner, we, as a wise person, who teaches the hungry person within our midst to fish rather than offering a fish to provide a single meal, teach clients and caregivers to self-sooth, which each and every one of us benefits from learning (Zukav, 1999). And we, as therapists, learn, through the use of negotiation as a partnering tool, to sharpen our listening skills and hone our speaking skills and to more deeply appreciate the reality that we are all more alike than we are different. That is what partnering helps impart to us.

3   WE ARE WHAT WE NEED

"I am enough. I do enough. I have enough."

--- Christiane Northrup, M.D., OB/GYN, Author

(Oprah Winfrey Show, October 16, 2007)

In the previous chapter, we reviewed a painfully humorous failed clinical encounter. The exchange took place between a robotic hospital grief liaison counselor and Richard Hoover, the dazed adult son of a freshly departed father, in the Oscar-nominated film in The Best Picture of 2006 category, *Little Miss Sunshine*. The counselor, increasingly enraged as Richard intensely probes the necessity of her time-consuming paperwork demands, resembles those of us who, deep within ourselves, cling to the battered and shredded belief that devoted service to our employer identifies us as the good employees we want to be known to be. When others appreciate our efforts with *kudos*, we feel validated. We feel happy. But, when they react to our work with indifference or, even, rejection, our self-worth plummets. We feel sad and hurt. We smart at being misunderstood. We rankle at the unfairness. At some point, saturated with these throbbing feelings, we direct our anger toward those we sincerely wanted to help, clients and caregivers and employers. We begin by convincing ourselves, *"No good deed goes unpunished."* We hold to the axiom, *"The tall grass gets mowed first."* We feel self-righteous. We seek the protection and revenge we feel we need and deserve. We stifle our zeal. We rein in our enthusiasm. We harden our hearts. Enmeshed in our own needs and fears, we fail to recognize or remember that clients and caregivers and employers pursue their own agendas and that their actions toward us may reflect unresolved conflicts with individuals for whom we may only be unwitting stand-ins (Please review "Projections" in Chapter 1.) And we also fail to recognize or recall that what we think of ourselves matters more than what others think of us.

The Avoidable Path to Burn-Out

Like the hapless hospital grief liaison counselor in *Little Miss Sunshine*, we may use our own hurt and angry feelings following work-related impasses to mistakenly convince ourselves that emotionally distancing ourselves from clients and caregivers will spare us further pain. But turning our emotional backs on clients and caregivers and employers eventually boomerangs. We provide a broader target for their dissatisfaction because we now appear cold and disinterested in their needs and concerns. And we pay a stiff price for depriving ourselves of our innate desire to deftly and skillfully touch and genuinely be touched by others' lives (Goleman, 2006). We become tired, depressed, and irritated. We have difficulty falling or staying asleep. We are too distracted to enjoy time with family and friends. We overeat and become increasingly sedentary or fanatically exercise and diet. We suffer from assorted bodily aches and pains. We rarely enjoy a hearty belly laugh. We find work boring and routine. We just go through the motions. We realize we are very unhappy. We try to mask our unhappiness by acting giddy and feel foolishly false. We are burning-out. And, so, tragically and ironically, by withdrawing emotionally to avoid pain, we cause ourselves anguish. We need to find a better way out. And we can. We only need look within.

SELF AWARENESS

If we prepare to contribute positively to others' lives, we have made a noble choice that will bring us unparalleled happiness. But, if we do the work to seek approval from clients, caregivers, colleagues, employers, and others so we can feel good, special, or, even, adequate, we suffer. We create a painful dilemma by seeking others' appreciation of our work to feel valued and worthwhile or to elevate our position in life. We may as well continue to believe in the jolly fellow in the red suit and white beard. If we believed that kindly soul rewarded good children with presents at Christmas when we were young, we may recall that after the excitement of unwrapping the packages he supposedly left, playing with the toys, modeling the clothes, and stuffing the gifts of paper money into our banks inevitably faded, we were no more certain we really were good than before he arrived when we wondered whether or not we merited a visit. Some undoubtedly felt relief just to have received gifts and gave no more thought to whether Santa thought we were bad or good. But some of us felt somehow, someway we fooled him. We realized he must not have known we sometimes lied about classmates to avoid being punished for our misdeeds, palmed an infantry soldier's ring from our brother's desk drawer to bask in its cachet as we showed it to our first grade classmates, fake-coughed so we could spit wads of stringy, hated asparagus into our paper napkins at dinner, and threatened our pesky younger sister with annihilation if she told on us one more time. So, within hours, Santa's presents failed to convince us we were good because we knew differently. And we wondered what he would do to us if he found out. Contemplating the possibility, our anxiety ballooned.

As adults, we discovered it was not just gifts from Santa that failed to make us feel worthy if we felt otherwise. The stuff we amassed, the vacations we took, the cars we drove, the friends and acquaintances we made also failed to make us feel we were worthwhile. In fact, they only made us feel worse. We wondered why. Our anxiety increased even more. Sometime later we were fortunate to learn the only one way we can feel worthwhile is to know we are.

Consequences of Seeking Others' Validation of our Worth

When we are students, we need to earn passing grades in coursework and *practica* and to establish relationships with professors, instructors, and clinical staff that lead to complimentary letters of recommendation to support our applications for admission to graduate programs and, later, employment. During our Clinical Fellowship Year and beyond, we need to satisfy our supervisors and meld our skills well with colleagues to satisfy employer expectations. All along the way, we face decisions that cumulatively establish or deny our feelings of self-worth and color the quality of our service. Here are two circumstances to consider carefully.

Clinical Decision-Making. Expecting *kudos* from others for what we have and what we have done as validation of our worthiness puts us on a circus ride where we go round and round and up and down and feel unsteady when we disembark. We get stymied deciding whether we're good enough, and, sadly, but not surprisingly, we become diminished in our capacity to help as we fill with self-doubt. We feel elated, we feel useful, and we feel worthwhile when Mrs. Anton assures us we have done wonders helping Tommy, her six-year-old retarded son, learn to count to 10. Another day, Mr. Franklin unexpectedly text mails us an hour before his scheduled therapy session that he is quitting. He reports he *". . . wants to stop stuttering not talk about stuttering."* We feel stunned and hurt that he chose this closed, impersonal way of expressing such an important decision instead of discussing his concerns with us, and we feel angry and offended he offered such a skewed version of his therapy experience to justify his decision. We feel worthless. We also feel scared wondering if he will sue us. The day before, Sue, our supervisor, commented about how pleased the medical director told her she is with our leadership at head injury team meetings. We beam. We feel confident. But this evening, only one couple attended the post-stroke support group we facilitate. Twenty-four patients and family members attended the first meeting two months earlier. Except for gradually falling attendance, feedback has been good. We feel disturbed. We are failing. And so it goes when we depend on clients and caregivers to validate our self-worth. When they are happy working with us, we feel capable. We are happy. When they criticize or reject our work, we feel unworthy. We are unhappy. Sometimes all of our clients will be pleased with our work. Sometimes none will. Most of the time, some will, and some will not.

If we depend on clients', caregivers', and colleagues' satisfaction with our work to establish our sense of self-worth, emotionally we will bounce up and down like a "Yo-Yo." And, professionally, we will experience confusion making clinical decisions because we will lack confidence in our judgment. That is when we easily can behave like the enabling parent who fails to make healthy food choices for her morbidly obese son because she does not want to risk his disapproval when she deprives him of the greasy foods he craves. When we care more about attending to our own feelings than carrying-out our responsibilities for those with whom we work, our clinical judgment suffers and so do we.

Playing Politics. The path to professional practice is one of relationship-building. As students, we benefit from establishing supportive relationships with university and college instructional and supervisory staff to qualify for letters of recommendation to graduate school that amplify our potential as caring, conscientious professionals and, later, as applicants for employment. As practicing professionals, we benefit from developing collegial relationships with staff and administration needed to adequately meet the needs of clients, caregivers, and students-in-training. That we rely on productive relationships to achieve our potential and help those in our charge do the same is a given. But the watchword in doing so is *Caution*.

Some consider the process of developing worksite relationships as playing politics, and it is political. We work at establishing allies while creating minimal or no enmity. Just like the professional politico's, we can play well or poorly. Playing well, we put the needs of present and future clients and caregivers before our own. Playing poorly, i.e., taking a false path to demonstrate self-worth, we cloud our perception of quality professional service and risk failing those in our charge and ourselves. In the school systems, university programs, clinics, hospital settings, home health agencies, and in skilled nursing facilities in which I have worked, I have seen politics played fast, fierce, and endlessly. Rehabilitation Directors and area managers bored with the intricacies of patient care and obsessed with accumulating personal power can establish work environments where therapists expend more energy relating to staff than to patients in order to survive. For example, in the outpatient rehabilitation program for young adults with traumatic brain injury where I worked as senior therapist and team leader for several years, the Program Director, a relatively inexperienced, excessively ambitious psychologist, was consumed with what he boasted to me was making the program" . . . *the flagship of my fleet.*" He devised elaborate schemata for diagnostic and clinical-decision making that he presented at innumerable, unwelcome noon-hour staff meetings. This caused staff to spend hours consulting with each other to decide how to meet the changing protocol demands, a task which surfaced as a surrogate for the primary task of meeting patient needs. The Director also established a pre-workday series of meetings devoted to his presentation of research findings, much of which had extremely limited clinical application. While such dedication to staff training and program protocol development and implementation might seem desirable, using the force of his personality to do so actually disrupted patient care. He failed to allow for input from seasoned, caring staff, thereby diminishing their morale and enthusiasm. And he unambiguously communicated meeting his requirements was primary. Few wanted to risk his ire by deviating from his elaborate protocols, which eventually were seen as short-sighted and impractical. Before he was relieved of his position, considerable staff time and energy was diverted from addressing patients' needs to satisfy his personal ambition. Although experienced staff almost immediately perceived the Director's true motivations and the naiveté of his plan, they played along to keep their jobs, a dilemma many of us face daily. Striking a compromise between maintaining our own ethical standards, which involves placing the patient's needs first, and meeting employer demands for grandiosity of service requires considerable thought and reflection.

Working at a job where we think we can make little difference, we are likely to stride the safe, unexposed route to safeguard our employment. We avoid being the tall grass mowed first. We do what is required. We follow the *"letter of the law."* We test, we treat, we consult following established procedures, and, maybe, we shift our focus to conduct research, where we also follow protocols that relieve us of any temptation to open our hearts. We operate from our heads. We measure. We count. We tell, but we do not really counsel because we lack comfort and skill working with feelings. Of course, graduate programs following the lead taken by the profession molds us into practioners of this short-sighted, *Big Head/Little Heart*, i.e., left-brain approach, to clinical service.[1] The possibility does exist due to ASHA's recently introduced Evidence Based Practice requirement (Gottsfred, 2008), that relating from the heart as well as the head, an approach already characterizing the practice of some, will become increasingly prevalent. In fact, lawyer and New York Bestselling author, Daniel Pink (2006), predicts that right-brained dominance is becoming the norm in business and personal life in the west because of our explosive need for convincing stories within which to place left-brain observations. That means the arts, in particular, will becoming increasingly important avenues to establishing satisfying lifestyles, with MFA's becoming more desirable than MBA's to a comfortable future.

Sometimes, working in an environment where numbers rule, we feel considerable pressure to go along with colleagues' choices that we are told will enhance the reputation of the department or team even though we favor an alternative. This encouraged collegial accord as a pattern can morph into focusing more time and energy on chumminess than addressing patient needs. We develop schedules for bringing treats. We intensely share information about family and social relationships. We celebrate each other's birthdays. We go clubbing and to bars after work. We begin to feel our primary job is getting staff to like us. We begin to think we have joined a high school clique (Wiseman, 2003).

Eventually, we tire of seeking others' approval. We realize trying to be like others muddies our sense of self-worth. I think I first began to understand this idea when I went ice skating for the first time when I was 10.

My best friend's grandfather drove the two of us to an indoor rink. I was excited about doing something new and different but scared, too. Typical of me, I wanted to skate right, whatever right was. Mildly apprehensive, after I strapped on the rented, moth ball-reeking figures skates, I hesitantly tottered down the slatted wooden ramp from the staging area toward the rink. The press of energized skaters propelled me forward and held me back at the same time as some pushed to quickly reach the rink while others hurried from it. The stench of wet, warm wool mittens caused me to hold my breath tight as I hobbled to catch up with my friend well ahead of me.

Moving through a gap between tall and thick bodies, I stepped onto the ice and instantly enjoyed a cool, moist breath before recognizing the need to move on. I could not see my friend to know where to head, but that didn't matter. I needed to skate. I tentatively moved one leg, then the other. And the oddest thing happened: My left leg slowly slid out to the left while the right leg just as slowly went right. I was heading into the splits. The only thing I could think of doing to avoid a midline rupture was to lurch forward to fall on my hands and knees.

Standing up, I deliberately pressed my feet firmly onto the ice and slowly wiggled each until both were side-by-side. Determined to glide around the rink, I moved my legs as I had done before with the same results. Perplexed, as I once again worked my way into a standing position, I was determined to discover why I my legs moved sideways instead of forward. Looking closely at the surface of the ice for the first time, I instantly discovered why: It was uneven and rutted. Each of my skates followed a groove someone else's skate had cut. I immediately recognized I would have to make my own grooves if I wanted to skate where I wanted to go. So, I placed my feet firmly on the ice, decided where I wished to go, focused on that direction, moved my legs, and got there!

Likewise, in life, we need to make our own way. Following others' grooves may not only get us where we do not want to go but even can cause us harm. It is like playing our opponent's game instead of our own. When we do, we are likely to lose. We certainly will not do our best.

From early childhood, I became enchanted with the notion that doing what you believed was right no matter what others said and did was *the* way to live. This belief was underscored after reading numerous biographies when I was eight, especially those of Nathan Hale and Thomas Edison. I was incredibly impressed with Hale's willingness to give his life for an ideal and Edison's steadfastness and his mother's as well. She never wavered in her belief of her son, who had been expelled from school because, according to his teacher, his head was too large for him to succeed. His mother taught him at home, and we all know what he accomplished. And we know what he said helped make that possible, *"Invention is 1% inspiration and 99% perspiration."* How much happier and helpful, how much more satisfied and effective we all can be when, when, instead of depending on acceptance from others, we, like composer, musician, arranger, and conductor, Quincy Jones can say, *"Not one drop of my self-worth comes from acceptance from others."* (*Charlie Rose*, PBS, January 16, 2007) because we, too, realize the only acceptance that matters comes from within.

As we come to know ourselves as we really are, we become keenly aware we are fine, or, in Transactional Analysis terms, O.K. That is when, if we are lucky, we begin to suspect that our conditioned beliefs, i.e., the way we have learned to perceive ourselves, others, and the world may be what actually brings us happiness and unhappiness. We discover we can examine our feelings to reveal those core beliefs, make necessary adjustments in our thinking, and genuinely help others *without being hampered by the motivation of doing so to validate our personal worth because we already are beginning to know we are precious just as we are* (Mipham, 2007), or perfect as Zen master Suzuki Roshi suggested addressing an audience at The San

Francisco Zen Center. He reportedly said, *"You are all perfect, and you need a little work."* (Chödrön, 2005c).

The Dalai Lama (2006) provides an extensive, accessible guide to the process of becoming self-aware. A contemporary *New York Times* best-seller, *The Secret* (Byrne, 2006), provides a clear, focused method based on a clear rationale for accelerating self-awareness. And Chapter 1 of this text offers a brief introduction to meditation practices and self-reflection, two essential tools for increasing self-awareness irrespective of method's suggested for that purpose. As we come to know our real selves, we find it natural to accept who and what we are. And, when se do, we no longer need to talk incessantly about ourselves as though others were simply foils for our needs. That, of itself, helps us place our attention on clients and caregivers to more effectively help them to better know themselves (Ahlskog, 2001).

SELF-ACCEPTANCE

There is a telling scene in the brilliant, powerful film, *Mean Girls* (2004), based on the book *Queen Bees and Wannabes* by Rosalind Wiseman (2003) where several members of a high school clique appraise their own physical appearance standing before a full length mirror. One sighs, *"My hairline is all wrong."* Another laments, *"My eyebrows don't arch right."* And so on. The new member of the group who, until the current semester had been home schooled in Africa, quietly studies their intense, personal, fault-finding. Stunned, she mumbles to herself, *"I thought you were only fat or thin. I didn't know there could be so much wrong with our bodies."* There isn't. But so many of us, concerned with being accepted, seem pre-occupied with aligning our physical appearance with whatever apparent media standard currently is in vogue. Some of us concentrate on eradicating our supposed behavioral flaws, such as a stutter, a lisp, the fear of making small talk, etc. Only a few of us, for example, Quincy Jones, recognize that acceptance starts within. If we don't accept ourselves, few will. And if we do, it doesn't matter who else does or doesn't.

When I was collecting speech samples of four-year-old boys for my doctoral dissertation from the University of Iowa to assess the generality of their disfluencies from one situation to another, I became acquainted with Charlie. He was one of the 10 boys I studied. I sampled his speech and that of the remaining nine boys at the University of Illinois, Urbana, Child Development Preschool (Silverman, 1970). Charlie used a variety of precise words to make sparkling contributions to class discussions and conversation with classmates and while asking and answering prosaic and ordinary questions. His manner was self-assured, even, dignified. He was popular and well-respected by other boys and girls and classroom personnel. No one, not even he, seemed concerned he frequently repeated words and parts of words three, four, or five times in a row and often interjected sounds such as *"um"* and *"er"* at the start or mid-way through his remarks. He exuded confidence communicating. As a young boy, he accepted himself just as he was.

By the time we are young adults, accepting ourselves as we seem to be challenges many of us. From exposure to pervasive media messages designed to make us feel wanting combined with distorted messages delivered by powerful caregivers, we have come to believe we must be perfect to be acceptable and that we are not perfect. We adopt a false image of ourselves as flawed beings. Yet, we retain a slim awareness of our natural goodness, which we notice when we spontaneously pull someone from the path of a car, chase down someone who ran off with another's purse, clear snow from an elderly neighbor's sidewalk, gaze with awe at a golden sunrise, feel reverence listening to a strong tenor sing *Ave Maria*, and so on. These experiences lead us to feel refreshed and recharged because we have experienced the truth of who we really are by noticing how we naturally respond to other people and the world around us. But, for most of us, this feeling of profound acceptance is transient and quickly submerged. We soon revert to our more deliberate, customary manner of being, fault-finding and conditional rejection. Yesterday, Valentine's Day, the day many give and receive diamonds as symbols of never-ending love, I marveled at how similar to this brilliant gemstone we all are. Like diamonds encrusted with earth elements when found, our true nature may be partially or totally eclipsed by the condensed debris of conditioned thoughts and habitual behaviors. Skillful, resourceful, and patient removal of this debris finally reveals who we truly are.

Until recently, what I saw when I observed myself was the accumulated garbage of conditioned thinking and habitual behavior stemming in large part from the vicious, unrelenting verbal abuse delivered by my parents beginning when I was four. Eventually their distorted messages resurfaced inside my head when I experienced happenstances resembling childhood memories. For instance, when I looked at myself in a mirror, I expected to see and saw someone fat and ungainly because my stepmother referred to me as *"big, fat tub of lard"* among other things. I was surprised several years ago looking at old photo's to see how thin I actually was as a child and teen. When, adopting my parents' judgmental approach to relating with others, I discovered what they would consider to be flaws in acquaintances' background or behavior, I heard the echo's of my father's rebuke of my choice of friends, *"I can't let her out; she attracts all the squirrels."* When I approached a new task, I feared failure because my father called me *"The Big Dummy."* And so it went. Despite being aware of my good academic performance and clinical skills, I considered myself unsuccessful, even after earning a doctorate, completing a post-doctoral fellowship, publishing numerous papers in professional journals, delivering many conference papers, and, even, becoming a tenured university professor, because they demeaned my early academic success by snarling when they reviewed my report cards, *"It's only book knowledge; anybody can read a book."*

We Are OK

I began to change the perspective of myself as a loser in life as I trained to become a Transactional Analysis (TA) therapist. A major tenet of TA theory that we are all O.K. was excruciatingly difficult for me to understand and was a stumbling block for many of my fellow trainees as well. At the time, I was not very good at dealing with apparent para-doxes. Being O.K. but believing treatment benefits us was difficult to reconcile. When I began studying Buddhist psychology years later, I encountered the Shakyamuni Buddha's rendering of the same message, namely that we all possess the essentials for living well, i.e., goodness, awareness, curiosity, love of the world and each other (e.g., Ray, 2003), and that being who we are means cultivating these qualities. That was when I became able to accept myself. Before then, my focus had been on my perceived flaws, of which there seemed to be no lack. I considered myself a mess I did not want to claim. With this more complete understanding of my true nature, I eagerly accepted my new, enlarged vision of myself and learned to live it.

Some of us decide to wait to accept ourselves until we have established ourselves as the person we wish to be, i.e., lost the weight, increased physical endurance, found a partner, become pregnant, become free of debt, etc. Some of our clients hold to that view, too. An example of this personal outlook surfaced as a helpful, spirited exchange online in the fall of 2006 among several speech therapists who subscribe to the American Speech-Language-Hearing Association SIDIV listserv. This special interest division serves those interested in fluency and fluency disorders by encouraging sharing of clinical and research information. A member posted a concern expressed by a client, a woman with a stuttering problem. The client wondered whether accepting her stuttering meant the same as being defeated by it. Most subscribers advocated that the therapist provide counseling for this woman to help her understand the difference between acceptance of her stuttering and being defeated by her stuttering. My own contribution was as follows (edited for brevity):

> *If we can assume that, as humans, we are inconstant, i.e., ever-changing, then it becomes so much easier to accept ourselves as we are momentarily and as changing entities. So, to accept myself as I am and to acknowledge that I will be changing, I can devote my energy to changing in the direction I wish.*
>
> *I experienced the value of this orientation when I committed to losing a significant amount of weight. I praised myself for deciding to undertake an activity that was in my best interest. I did not hate myself because I was fat, which did take some doing. I loved myself for valuing myself and being willing to carry on in ways that were good for me. Not accepting oneself or a part of oneself ultimately causes major impediments to personal growth.*
>
> *Carl Jung, in his writings on the shadow element of the conscious self, wrote about the necessity of identifying and integrating the shadow to achieve wholeness. Self-acceptance becomes easier for us all when we recognize we are more than our personalities.*

So many of us defer accepting ourselves until we accomplish some future personal goal instead of accepting ourselves as we are each moment that *Greatest Love of All* released by singer Whitney Huston in 1986 struck a nerve in many, making it a huge hit by asserting, *"Learning to love yourself. It is the greatest love of all."*

When we accept ourselves for who we are, we can more readily accept others for who they are. Likewise, when we accept ourselves, we are much more able to move in the direction we desire rather than succumbing to a self-created climate of personal sabotage and defeatism, and we are much more able to help others accept themselves and go on to achieve their goals.

SELF-CONFIDENCE

The Elevation Effect

When we accept our true selves, we radiate a profound self-confidence that implicitly raises the *ante*. We subliminally encourage those around us to be and do their best. That is considered one of the greatest assets of legendary, record-breaking quarterback Brett Favre, who, because he believes he can win the game he is in, is known to elevate the play of his teammates. The New York Jets, the team he joined in 2008, compiled a dismal 4-12 record in 2007. In 2008, they established a winning record that makes them a strong contender for the playoffs (e.g., Pedulla, 2008). Isn't that what we all can do when we believe in ourselves? Conversely, when we deny our inherent intelligence, awareness, curiosity, and warmth because we are riddled by fear and doubt, we bring others down. We and they go flat. That is one essential reason self-acceptance is so important for us all. Without self-acceptance, we can not experience self-confidence. We might pretend to be self-confident, but without self-acceptance, we probably will project arrogance and, possibly, intolerance, and we will, at least temporarily, block progress, our own and our clients'.

One of the times most of us temporarily lack self-confidence is when we begin clinical work. For example, I received a post from a graduate student to a paper I presented at the 9th Annual International Stuttering Awareness Day (ISAD) Online Conference in 2006 expressing her anxiety about beginning clinical work. Like so many students, including me and my friends, her studies initially convinced her there was more to learn than she felt capable of knowing at the time she began providing treatment, and she recognized that she did not have all the direct, personal experience with self-change she hoped to have somewhat later in her life. I advised her as follows:

> *Dear Alyssa,*
>
> *I appreciate the thoughtful consideration you gave to what I had to say in "Mind Matters;" I felt your sincerity come through your words. And I have no doubt that the clients you work with from the beginning, and throughout your career, will be aware of your sincere desire to be of help to them. To be somewhat uncertain of*

oneself at the beginning of a career in speech therapy is not unusual at all. It was that way for me and for my fellow students. In fact, some of that uncertainty about how to work with a client is present each time I meet with a new one, and I suspect, for me at least, that is a very good thing because it prevents me from being rote and robotic in my work. But, like everything else, balance is important. The client is appreciative and more open to change with a therapist who appears confident so much so that he or she can attend carefully to them because he or she is not burdened by concerns about how well they are doing what they are doing. That doesn't mean that he or she knows all the answers to every inevitability but that he or she knows how to find the answers for himself or herself. Key personal qualities to being a helpful therapist,

I believe, are compassion, kindness, and friendliness. I also believe being able to listen well is very important. Then it is critical to recognize the client as a colleague in the process and to foster mutuality from the very beginning in regard to goal selection, methods used, timelines, etc.

I would say to you that instead of investing your energy in your anxiety about not being helpful enough you should consider learning what you think you need to know and what you want to know about disorders, about clinical skills, and about yourself. Self-knowledge is precious for so many reasons, one of which is that the better we know ourselves, the better we can know others. So, you want to build your knowledge and skill base, which you will do throughout your career, and your confidence, which you also will build throughout your career and life. Based on my experience, working with each new client is an adventure and an opportunity to learn something new. That could be about communication problems, clinical skills, and/or yourself. Release yourself from the concern you do not know enough since you do not know that you do not know enough! If you are determined to do so, and you seem to be, you will learn what you need to know, and you will help your clients, do the same IF they are truly open to learning and doing the necessary work to do so   As we learn to monitor our feelings, behavior, and intent; accept ourselves for the gifted, splendid beings we are; and reflect the self-confidence that arises from such self-knowledge, we know incontrovertibly we have all we need to do what we need to do and to do that well.

4   UNDERSTANDING TRUMPS KNOWING

"A cynic is a man who knows the price of everything and the value of nothing."

- - - Oscar Wilde

Reportedly, a sign on one of Albert Einstein's Princeton University office walls proclaimed,

"Some things that can be counted don't count,

and some things that count can't be counted."

I think many of us believe that. Yet, we tend to outwardly cave to collegial pressure to put a premium on information we gather by quantifying what we can easily and readily measure. In the process, we accumulate a mass of numerical data and sometimes wonder what real good that does for our clients. That is a very good question. It gets us thinking about how to measure, rather than ignore, the meaningful, seemingly, immeasurables, such as existential beliefs (e.g., Spillers, 2007), that we believe contribute significantly to clients' and caregivers' well-being (e.g., Simon, 2008) yet shy away from assessing. And, then, we begin to truly be of service.

SIX DEGREES OF KEVIN BACON

Many of us have played the *Six Degrees of Kevin Bacon* game that began on college campuses in the '90's. Based on the so-called *small world phenomenon*, the object is to connect actors to Kevin Bacon as quickly, and with as few links, as possible. Discovering the hundreds and thousands of actors sharing linkages with Mr. Bacon is a lot of fun. Growing up Jewish in the '50's, I witnessed my parents, their relatives, and their adult friends play a more insular version of the game called *Jewish Geography*. Two or more teens or adults who are strangers become the players. They seek to identify people they know in common to establish an immediate connection. One player might begin as follows:

Sam:*"Where are you from?"*

Aaron:*"Illinois. Champaign-Urbana."*

Sam:*"Champaign-Urbana? Do you know Mabel Schwartz?*

She's a bookseller there."

Aaron (with delight):*"Yes. My Aunt Sylvia bought books*

from her for years. I've been to her shop. It's in

the Lincoln Mall."

The premise is that if we can discover someone we know in common, we will feel less anxious and more willing to relate, and the common bond, no matter how tenuous, provides a context within which to begin. But this ice-breaker can reduce the way we relate to instant stereotyping. When someone plays the game with me and discovers a personal connection, I generally feel annoyed rather than pleased by their self-congratulatory smiles, frowns, winks, or other gestures and statements such as, *"Oh, I know her. She was married to Finch."* that immediately follow. Collectively, they imply I am now *kosher* by association, no longer the feared, possibly loathsome, stranger of Jewish lore. I now own membership in the gang and presumably share the goals, beliefs, and values of its members. I am someone safe.

I do not feel elated by this attribution. I feel slimed, slathered with gooey, improbable, bogus assumptions and presumptions of who I am that almost always encourage a forced, instant, one-sided intimacy. I do not feel known or understood, nor do I want to be by someone so apparently crass. I quickly retreat. Maybe I need more coping skills. Maybe I need better coping skills. Maybe I'm a snob, but I do not choose to relate socially to someone I consider so ignorant and insensitive.

Yet, I recognize one of my deepest, most compelling needs is to feel understood by someone close to me. Like most of us, I do not want to journey through life alone. So I keep looking for my identical psychic twin, who I believe, once found, surely and readily will know and understand me, but the more I look, the more I realize it is I who I need to understand me. I see that as I do, I become less vulnerable to exploitation by those who would use my longing to manipulate me into serving their needs while neglecting my own. And I feel more joyful and satisfied as I live an increasingly full life securely standing on my own two feet. Unlike Blanche DuBois, the mentally fragile character in Tennessee Williams' play, <u>A Streetcar Named Desire</u>, who proclaimed, *"I have always depended on the kindness of strangers,"* then was institutionalized after being raped by her brother-in-law and betrayed by her sister, I now choose to depend upon myself. As an interesting twist on trusting others, psychologist Dr. Phillip McGraw asserts: *When we believe we can handle whatever life brings, we do not need to live in fear that others may not take care of us.*

Clients

Clients, young and old, verbal and non-verbal, and their caregivers share the same primal need to be known and understood. Relating with us, they, no more than I playing "Jewish Geography," want to be seen as the unique human beings they believe themselves to be, not as: The Dysarthric. The Stutterer. The Child With Asperger's Syndrome. The Cleft Palate. The TBI. The Aphasic's Wife. The Teen With ADHD. Or any other stereotype. They want to be known as people, not things to be prodded, tested, and trained. They know when we perceive them as things instead of people, we cruelly limit their opportunity to rise. We cage them. And, if we look deeply at the effects of relating coldly and stereotypically, we see it diminishes us as well. We become less likely to help heal because we lack the particular insights and knowledge we would gain by fearlessly relating to clients as the individuals they are. Our job satisfaction suffers. Our effectiveness declines. Our personal life suffers because we feel energetically drained by working without fulfillment. Burn-out becomes a distinct possibility (Charon, 2006). This becomes our lot because we distanced ourselves from our clients and caregivers to focus on their problems instead of who they are in a misguided effort to be efficient and effective. And so, ironically, we heighten our risk of rejection and failure.

Two clients abandoned health care situations where, in their words, staff related to them *"as a piece of meat."*

> *Mike, a police officer, who suffered traumatic brain damage after crashing his car during high-speed motor vehicle chase, strenuously complained his speech therapist "pushed him around," saying, "Do this. Do that." He told her he wanted to be included in all aspects of decision-making but said she was not interested in partnering with him. She only seemed to care about her performance and concentrated on counting, measuring, and timing his responses to seemingly esoteric tasks, so he quit (Silverman, 2003a).*

> *Victor, suffering from a degenerative disease of the central nervous system, briefly became a patient at a nursing home where I worked for a short time. Relatives transferred him to this facility from an out-of-state nursing home where he longingly reported that nursing and rehabilitation staff cared about him as a person. Victor angrily complained about his care there. He said that the nurses seemed more concerned about changing his position, feeding, medicating him, and counting his bowel movements than about him as a person. From my perspective, he was correct. Within two weeks, he convinced his family to transfer him to a different facility.*

Because they long to be understood, clients and caregivers resist being related to as objects of pity even when they solicit sympathy. Early in my private practice while a university professor, I provided voice therapy to 50-something Arnie, who tapped deeply into my compassionate nature.

> *Arnie claimed prolonged laryngeal intubation several months earlier for cardiac surgery created contact ulcers on the medial surfaces of his arytenoid cartilages stripped him of the clear and strong voice he needed to continue his practice as a trial attorney. He claimed to be devastated by his now professionally ineffective and, he feared, unalterable, voice so he initiated litigation against the anesthesiologist who performed the intubation to obtain compensation for the pain, suffering, and income loss abandoning an established practice brought him.*

> *During our third or fourth weekly session, I introduced a conversational topic I believed would interest him as I audio-taped his voice. He spoke passionately and vocalized normally for several consecutive seconds until he became aware he was producing a completely functional voice. He abruptly stopped speaking, demanded to return to the vocal exercises he had been practicing, and never returned, although he failed to directly inform me then or later that he was ending treatment.*

In hindsight, I recognize he worked hard to tap into my compassionate nature to encourage me, a university professor, to take him as a client solely to help bolster the merits of his case since he planned for the therapy to be unsuccessful. From then on, I decided to scrupulously examine the motives of potential clients actively litigating for pain, suffering, and financial loss resulting from a problem for which they sought my help. Arnie's behavior helped teach me that clients seeking sympathy are clients handing out invitations to play The Rescue Dance (See Chapter 2), an opportunity the forewarned therapist wisely side-steps or risks the potential of feeling like road kill by a revenge-seeking, anger-blinded, or opportunistic client.

Many clients, however, behave as Sr. Anne by firmly refusing sympathetic responses we may, otherwise, generously apply to them. Sr. Anne, an inpatient rehabilitation client I worked with one morning while substituting for her customary staff speech therapist, suffered traumatic brain injury after a fall down a convent stairway. Shortly after noticing me silently pitying her while watching her struggle in the small bathroom of her hospital room to relearn basic self-care skills modeled by a staff occupational therapist, she sternly, clearly, and stunningly warned me, *"I need empathy, not sympathy!"* Those words were the first she uttered weeks after her accident. Until that moment, staff considered the silent sister globally aphasic![1] Sr. Anne, wise woman that she was, probably made the effort to say what she said because she knew I needed to hear that relating to a patient as someone deserving sympathy sabotages their growth while relating empathetically encourages it (Silverman, 2003a).

Once we set our mind to relating empathetically and compassionately, we realize we need to attend well (Shafir, 2000).

FULL-BODY ATTENDING

Attending Encourages Healing

We know the importance of listening well. When we listen attentively, we can hear and, perhaps, remember what is said. Listening well not only secures information it conveys respect. By offering our attention to another, we validate that individual by implicitly stating, *"Of all the activities I could engage with in this moment, I have chosen to relate to you."*

That is why the role of listening plays such a critical role in relationships, personal and professional. The act of listening well says, *"I am there for you. I will do my best to see that you have what you need to grow and flourish."* Listening well is an act of love that validates life itself. Placing us squarely in the moment, attentive listening demonstrates our appreciation of life by our willingness to actively respond to the gifts it brings moment-by-moment rather than denying its preciousness through worry and regret. Listening well encourages healing. Rabbi Yosef Samuels of the Milwaukee *Chabad* and teacher of *Torah* and *Kabbalah* believes we provide immeasurable relief to one another by the act of listening attentively to each other's concerns. The level of listening that communicates the respect, encourages the sharing of valuable information, and provides the relief that can help change peoples' lives involves the focused application and integration of several sensory activities: hearing, seeing, and sensing. These three activities can be artfully combined into one I call *full-body attending* through skilled interpretation and integration of that which is observed both inside and outside our seemingly personal space.

Hearing

Jack Kornfield (2003) related the story about an indigenous people. This poignant tale may or may not be true. I would like to believe it is.

> *When a woman of the tribe wanted to bear a child, she trekked to an area apart from her village to sit beneath a particular tree. She sat under the tree until she heard the song of the child waiting to be born to her. After she learned the song, she returned to the tribe and taught it to her partner. Then, when they made love, they sung the song together to invite the child to be born to them. When the woman knew she was pregnant, she taught the song to the midwife so she could sing the song to welcome the child into this world. Later, all members of the tribe learned the child's song and sung it when the child needed comforting and at rites of passage, such as marriage ceremonies, when the two partners' songs were sung. Then, finally, when the child left this earth, members of the tribe gathered to sing the song as a final, loving 'Good-Bye.'*

How wonderful to live in a community where we care enough to learn each other's songs and, of course, our own. Of course, few of us do. We race around over-booked, taking classes, working, carving out careers, and caring for partners, family members, pets, friends, homes, and cars. We rarely take time to deeply attend to ourselves and each other. We are too busy and too fatigued. And so we feel alone, even with intimates. That is why we so appreciate knowing someone who listens well.

Rachel Stuart, an attendee at Hillary Rodham Clinton's Conversations with Voters in Berlin, New Hampshire, in March, 2007, responded favorably to the Democratic Party candidate for President in 2008, because she listened to those present. Ms. Stuart was quoted as saying,

"She connected with me much better than I expected she would. She was right there. There was a real sense of her as a great listener (Leibovich, 2007)."

Ms. Stuart connected with Mrs. Clinton because she appeared present. She was right there. She seemed genuinely responsive rather than mechanical. She looked the person in the eye whose hand she shook. She asked questions of the individuals who came to meet her and nodded often while quietly listening to their replies. She maintained her focus on the individuals she met, singly and as a group. That quality of being present is the *sine quo non* of listening well. As a good, even great, listener, we are *right there*. We attend as long as it takes. We do nothing else except, perhaps, breathe. We do not text-message, check e-mails, worry, wonder what's for dinner, hope the mechanic finally has satisfactorily fixed our car's ignition problem, or do anything but concentrate on the person with whom we expect to communicate. We can try to convince ourselves we can successfully listen while multi-tasking because we recall words that were said and accompanying feelings and some thoughts seemingly associated with them, but when we put callers on speakerphone so we can write checks as they talk, enter data in the computer while a student asks a question about the class lecture we delivered yesterday, review our personal calendar while attending a staff meeting, we surely will not give the impression we are validating the one speaking or the one to whom we are speaking.

Validation is what most of our clients seek from us. They expect us to know what they have said and to recognize and acknowledge their feelings, i.e., empathize with them, if we expect them to partner with us. We need to quietly listen without judgment or expectation to what they say and how they say it as well as what they do not say.

To do that, we focus on who is addressing us and to our internal responses while we do. We maintain a relaxed awareness as we listen to what they say, how they say it, and what they seem to leave unsaid. We note their accompanying facial and body language. And, simultaneously, we note alterations in our breathing pattern and shifts in muscular tension throughout our physical body (e.g., Ray, 2003). We also note and consider whatever mental images, sounds, and, infrequently, smells accompany what we hear and note in our bodies.

Seeing

"We don't see things as they really are. We see things as we are."

- - - Anais Nin, writer, diarist

When we observe people, places, animals, sculpture, scenic vistas, weather or other phenomena or read newspapers, novels, journal articles, textbooks or other textual material, we interpret what we see. In a sense, we have no other choice. All such objects are empty of meaning. It is we who must assign their meaningfulness to us or else drift through life. For instance, when we notice a particular chair, we will consider it primarily as comfortable or uncomfortable or something in-between if we are tired and looking for a place to sit. If we are taking a course in design, we may consider that same chair primarily as artful, common-place utilitarian, or something in-between. And, if we are in need of extra cash, we may consider that very same chair primarily as a potential income source. Yet the chair is the chair is the chair. It hasn't changed, but as our needs and interests vary, we view it differently. In fact, we may not notice the chair at all if we weren't looking for a place to sit, or considering the design of objects, or driven by the need to obtain money.

I believe Dean Williams was the first to acquaint me with the notion that nothing we see has any meaning except that which we attach to it. Dean, who served as my thesis and, later, my dissertation advisor, at the University of Iowa, repeatedly reproached my writing of the results section of my thesis because I thought simply presenting the data in lists and tables was sufficient. Dean insisted, *"Data don't say what they mean. You have to say what they mean."* He taught me my job was to use them to make sound clinical decisions. About that time, in a *duh* moment, I began to notice that was what we as clinicians rarely do. We make decisions based more on subconsciously held beliefs and stereotypes about our client's appearance than on the actual interview and test data we compile from testing. Research describing the clinical decision-making process physicians' use (e.g., Groopman, 2007) shows they, too, are strongly influenced by a client's appearance. We know how strongly appearance influences the way we relate to one another. Media personalities donning fat suits receive rude and hurtful comments and taunts when they appear grossly obese in public. The Golden Globe award winning television comedy *Ugly Betty* that originated in Columbia, South America, exposes our obsession with appearance, as do the films, *Mean Girls* (2004) and *Shallow Hal* (2001). Novels do so even more. By excluding the distraction of appearance, they encourage us to attune our attention to the thoughts and intentions of the various assorted characters. Perhaps, because we become acquainted with them through consideration of their character, we refer to them as *characters*. As we become absorbed in the way they think, we relate to and learn from those of genders and ages different from our own, and we do so more readily than if we could see them before us. We become wizened from these vicarious experiences with diverse family and social encounters, financial circumstances, political affiliation and ideology, geographic and historical setting, sexual behavior, cultural influences, etc. we might, otherwise, either have missed or avoided. Yet, because of our preoccupation with visual appearance, when we hear that a novel will be translated into film, we hunger to see how the characters will look.

Our Fixation with Appearance

Our fixation with appearance is why many of us spend considerable time and money to look youthful, fit, and well-off. Perhaps, that is why elementary and middle school children, who are keen observers of what we do and say, are showing early symptoms of eating disorders typically diagnosed during adolescence. As therapists, we are not immune from society's influences nor are we unresponsive to our personal biases about each other. For instance, a therapist might withhold treatment from someone appearing homeless if the therapist believed homeless individuals were too unreliable to benefit from therapy while another might decide to provide treatment for the very same individual based on their belief that a marginalized client might be highly motivated to do what was required to become more integrated into mainstream society. Another therapist might predict a middle age male wearing his hair in a pony tail would experience a less favorable therapy outcome for vocal hygiene intervention than an adolescent boy wearing a sport coat and tie, while believing a middle-aged male bank executive might experience a more successful outcome for a similar intervention program than an adolescent boy sporting body piercing and spiked orange hair, even when testing yielded identical findings regarding all four hypothetical individuals.

What we believe trumps what we observe. We draw on our beliefs to decide what help, if any, we will offer clients and caregivers and how we will offer it, and few of us know that is what we do. *Why?* Because the beliefs that drive our decision-making personally and professionally generally reside in our unconscious. We may not know we have them until and unless someone cares enough to suggest that we do. Only when we bring them into our awareness, can we be assured we will be as helpful to ourselves and others as we could. The following three scenarios each report actual and divergent clinical decisions regarding the treatment of clients I and my colleagues have made. They, like most key decisions, express personal beliefs deeply held.

Example 1

When I was a university professor in the early to mid-'70's, a popular, young sports broadcaster from our local ABC affiliate applied to our speech clinic for a speech evaluation and therapy, if necessary.

He worried he lisped, and he was concerned that if he did and did not stop, the might be jeopardizing his broadcasting career. While all members of the faculty and clinical staff except the lone audiologist were certified speech-language pathologists, none wanted to evaluate him. They seemed intimidated by his local star status. I, being fearless in that respect, volunteered to evaluate his speech and did.

Example 2

Also, in the late '70's, an investment banker contacted our speech clinic to apply for a voice evaluation. Burt, a 30-ish transgender person preparing to live the following year as his female identified self, Roberta, wished to develop a speaking voice appropriate for Roberta. Since I taught the voice disorders class, the clinic secretary logically placed him on my clinic schedule. I had some apprehension about working with Burt/Roberta[2] since I, like most speech therapists at the time, had little knowledge about transgender individuals as clients and no experience meeting their oral communication needs. And, more fundamentally, as someone with a long-standing fear of sweeping personal change, I was mildly unsettled about the possibility of partnering with someone committed to altering their gender to recalibrate and rearrange their entire life. But, simultaneously, as someone who has always sought high personal challenges, I found the opportunity to help Burt/Roberta live a fulfilling life extremely compelling. .My department colleagues, including the chair, at this conservative Catholic university were not sympathetic with my decision to evaluate Burt/Roberta and to provide voice therapy as needed. The afternoon Burt/Roberta arrived to be evaluated, several staff remained in the clinic building long after they ordinarily would have left for the day. They conspicuously loitered throughout the clinic to observe Burt arrive, dress himself as Roberta, and walk to my office. The following day, prior to the convening of our weekly department faculty meeting, several muttered among themselves loudly enough for me to hear that they wouldn't waste their time working with a "freak."

Example 3

When I worked for a very short while in a county owned, long-term nursing facility local residents nicknamed "Pill Hill," I learned that Pat, a charge nurse in one of the units was, as the experienced occupational therapist described, "anti-therapy." I soon discovered that, like many RN's at the facility, Pat referred patients for therapy evaluation and treatment only when it served her particular need to demonstrate through documentation that she did what was necessary to provide required patient care. Yet she brazenly disregarded occupational and physical therapy and speech therapy recommendations for follow-through activities to be carried out on the unit.

I met with Pat one morning to review swallow safety recommendations I had made the prior week for Mrs. Albert, a patient on her unit. I had reason to believe the guidelines had not yet been put into place since the nursing staff had sent her to speech therapy the previous day clutching a partially eaten banana. I reminded Pat that if staff did not implement those procedures with Mrs. Albert when she ate and drank, they would be placing her at high risk for aspiration pneumonia and choking. Pat proudly and defiantly replied, "I have no trouble with patients dying. I'm not afraid of death."

Each of the decisions I made as a service provider stemmed from one of my core beliefs about working as a therapist, namely, to be of service to all who seek my assistance. Of course, we can only surmise what my colleagues' underlying personal beliefs may have been that triggered their decisions. I suspect that if I had asked them what they were, they may have been incredulous at being asked and probably either unable to say or embarrassed to do so. Nevertheless, the following may be quite close to the mark.

> For Example 1: *Me First - I Prefer to Work with Less Powerful*
>
> *People.*
>
> For Example 2: *Don't Become Tainted by Offering Services*
>
> *to People Outside Society's Mainstream.*
>
> AND
>
> For Example 3: *To Hell With Life When You Are Old and Infirm.*

These real-life examples demonstrate how stereotypes and beliefs can drive our clinical decision-making. Knowing that, wisdom dictates that we take to heart the advice Socrates and other sages offered healers long ago, i.e., *"Know thyself."*

A key element of knowing ourselves is recognizing our core beliefs (e.g., H.H. the Dalai Lama, 2006). From years of self-reflection, I have learned deep self-knowledge becomes possible when we are attuned to what we think, feel, and do *in the moment*. This awareness is both purpose and reward of an ongoing *mindfulness* or *insight meditation practice* (e.g., Hahn, 2004; Kabat-Zinn, 2005, 2006; Kornfield, 1998; Salzberg and Goldstein, 2002) and certain variations, such as *shenpa practice* (e.g., Chödrön, 2005b; Silverman, 2005), Mindfulness Based Stress Reduction (MBSR) developed and taught by Jon-Kabat Zinn (2005) and those he has trained, and the practice of challenging personal beliefs labeled The Work and taught by Byron Katie (e.g., 2003). Research shows (e.g., Tuma, 2007) practices such as these help us train our minds to become calm, steady, and focused so we can look deeply within to locate, excavate, and examine our core beliefs and to calmly and surely respond to stimuli from without. The time required to establish and maintain such a practice may be as few as 10 consecutive minutes daily (e.g., Mipham, 2006). By consistently and patiently committing to a practice, we slowly but surely deepen in our understanding of ourselves and others. The results can be quite subtle at first. We might, for example, think we have not accomplished anything. Yet we become aware that colors seem more vivid, that aromas and odors scent the air, that people are more interesting, that music has more depth, that we have fewer accidents, etc. This is an early fruit of the practice. Our mind is becoming steady. Instead of flitting about here and there and everywhere dragging our attention along with it, it is becoming more focused more of the time.

Basic instruction can be obtained from a variety of textual (e.g., Hahn, 2000; Katie, 2003), audio (e.g., Chödrön, 2006: Hanh, 2004; Katie, 2007; Ray, 2003), video (e.g., Kornfield, 1998), and or various combinations of these media forms (e.g., Kornfield, 1998; Kornfield, 2001; Kabbat-Zinn, 20021) and, of course, from private instruction and/or attendance at classes, workshops, and retreats. I began my practice in earnest (Silverman, 2003d) while experiencing a crisis of spirit. Certainly, we do not have to wait for a crisis to discover who we are and to live authentically. We can join the estimated 10 million children and adults in the United States of America (Stein, 2003; Tuma, 2007) who meditate daily following practices based on secular and non-secular foundations. Take the time to select the practice best suited to you. Then begin. Reading about meditating and talking about meditating and thinking about meditating is not meditating.

Mind Over Matter. When we set a goal and focus our energies on meeting it, we follow a mind over matter approach to life. We may use our supple minds to select and chart a path to create a sustainable planetary environment, become a billionaire-philanthropist, run successfully for a seat in Congress, increase our self-awareness, or realize any other goal we find compelling. My first Transactional Analysis trainer insisted that, in this life, we either control or are controlled. I can accept her assertion when I define control as self-control. When we become self-directing, we diminish the likelihood others, usually parents, partners, employers, members of the same faith community, politicians, and organizations and corporate entities, can successfully manipulate us into behaving how they wish in order to realize their desires, goals, and wishes (e.g., Mipham, 2006). Some friends, family, or acquaintances believing we have set our mind on obtaining a goal they fear will separate us from them and reduce their influence on us will try to discourage us from making the commitment or cast us aside. For instance, my father's and stepmother's families, which always demanded complete allegiance of its members, essentially cast me and my daughter aside when we became vegetarians in 1981, the only family members who were. The rest stopped inviting us to family gatherings. The reason they gave was, *"We don't know what to serve you."* Even though I assured them there was no need to make special provisions for us because there always would be enough food we for us to eat well and be satisfied, they remained unrelenting.

Those who fear their status in the family or community may diminish or their self-concept may suffer or we may abandon them if they do not accomplish what we might also try to sabotage our efforts. Those individuals often attempt to dismiss our goals as folly. They may speak disparagingly to us and to those we know who they consider influential about the questionable value of our goals or our limited capacity to achieve them. To us, they sometimes dismiss our efforts as *"nothing more than mind over matter,"* as if they take no effort whatsoever to accomplish and, as such, reflect no hard-won achievement of which to be proud or, even, satisfied, and certainly not to be recognized for, all in an effort to keep their status, self-concept, and relationship with us from changing.

Recently, a reader of the paper I presented at the 2006 International Stuttering Awareness Day (ISAD) Conference, Mind Matters, chided me for writing that approaching stuttering therapy with a *mind over matter attitude*, as Tiger Woods apparently did as a young child, can lead to a successful therapy outcome like his. She made the following post:

"Do you really believe that overcoming stuttering is as simple as mind over matter?"

To which, I replied:

". . . let me say that "mind over matter" is not simple. For those attempting to change their beliefs and behaviors, it is quite the opposite. Learning to slow down enough to observe one's thoughts, feelings, and behaviors without judgment but with kindness toward oneself so one wants to continue the process of change, which never runs smoothly but occasions set-backs small and large, requires commitment, perseverance, and patience. That said, let me now say that those very activities are central to changing. If a person says they want to change their stuttering behavior, then, in my opinion, this is what is required. How else can change be brought about without self-observation, self-reflection, and the substitution of new beliefs and new behaviors for those which do not support functioning as desired? I know only that if we want to change, we must change. That means thinking differently and acting differently."

Approaching a goal with a mind over matter orientation does not guarantee achieving that goal, but the total experience can be positive. The discipline developed can lead to deeper personal insights and understanding of how to live well. And the process itself can lead to opportunities for personal happiness, contentment, peace, and material well-being that, otherwise, may not surface, at least for a time.

Sensing

Several days ago, I had an appointment with a physician who did not know me from personal experience or through acquaintance with my medical records, which were not fully accessible since I had not visited a physician in the facility for more than seven years. In the opening 5-10 minutes of our session, he asked predictable, basic questions relative to my health history and my present situation and firmly advised me to undergo routine examination and testing. As he was exiting, seemingly as an after thought, he turned toward me. Extending his right hand, he said, *"Let's see what kind of grip you have. Squeeze. Hard."* I did, delighted to have the chance to make the point that while I may have difficulty walking, I had no other musculoskeletal problems. Grinning, as he withdrew his hand from what I proudly imagined was a vise-like grip, he remarked admiringly that I was strong. Wanting to deflect his complement to disconnect from him, I replied, *"I have a 50 pound dog I need to handle."* He smiled for the second time and, eyes twinkling while staring firmly and knowingly into mine, remarked, *"He leads you around more than you know!"* He was spot on correct! I confirmed that to him with a quasi-conspiratorial smile of momentary, situational relationship. He returned the smile in kind, a pleasant closure to an otherwise uncomfortable experience.

I dote on that Basenji-mix dog to the extent others have warned me I was spoiling him. How this physician accurately perceived the nature of my relationship with Hansom, my animal companion of nine years, had to be attributed to his highly developed intuitive sense, which I had not suspected. He was intuitively skilled enough to perceive my inclinations and propensities so that when I mentioned I cared for a dog he correctly gauged an essential element of the relationship. That he shared that insight confirmed his desire to relate, for what purpose was not entirely clear. Nevertheless, a physician so attuned to me and willing to relate is the only one I would consider as a personal physician. I certainly would not choose someone who was not, who perceived me only as a collection of body parts and systems to be measured, manipulated, and medicated.

Many years ago, I first began to incorporate intuition into my clinical work in part because a friend, Corrine, a physician, shared she relied on her intuitive sense as a sound, reliable, clinical tool. As an example, she told me that recently she left the hospital where she practiced radiology-oncology to return home for the evening. Driving home, she sensed the need to go back to the hospital immediately. That was a time in recent history when cell phones were not available or possibly, even, imagined, and pagers were uncommon. Having had enough experience with her intuition, she unhesitatingly turned her car around. When she arrived back at her office, she learned a young female patient of hers needed urgent care. Because she had followed her intuition, she was able to oversee the successful handling of what she believed was a menacing crisis. I think Corrine knew sharing that experience would help free me from a deep personal conflict embroiling me.

Enrollment in the graduate program where I earned a master's and a Ph.D. that was staffed by fiercely committed behavioral scientists placed me in severe conflict with honoring my intuition, which, through hunches and insight had shown me what to believe from childhood on. To survive in that circumstance, I took the low road: I conformed. I turned off my intuition to rely on objective evidence instead. I decided that was easier and safer than defending hunches to the seemingly left-brained faculty that seemed to hold my future in their hands. But lopping off such a basic part of me, which included joy and mystery, had catastrophic consequences. Even though, I spent slightly less than four years in the department, three on-site, the training took. I, too, functioned as a behaviorist, proudly defining, counting, and measuring rather than deeply attending. After more than 10 years without the energizing effect of intuition as guide, I was languishing. And I knew it. By the time I had come to know Corrine, I was almost empty of drive, enthusiasm, satisfaction, and humor. My eyes appeared lifeless. I was barely present. After coming to admire how integrated, energetic, robust, and "tuned-in" she seemed, I wanted to be as she, in fact, as I remembered myself being. But, when I thought of returning to pre-graduate school me, I found myself mired in conflict between recovering what I had forgone to face probable rejection from my statistician husband blinded to beauty or remaining in the tight little box where I resided becoming increasingly lifeless.

Corrine's sharing pushed me off the proverbial fence. Her disclosure followed by acquaintance with the outstanding, and, even, seminal work of physicians-authors-teachers, such as Eric Berne (1977), Larry Dossey (2006; 1998), Christiane Northrup (2005), Judith Orloff (2004), C. Norman Shealy (1988), Mona Lisa Schulz (2005), Bernie Siegel (1986), and, of course, Elisabeth Kubler-Ross (1997), based, in part, on their intuition has helped keep me off. That learning, coupled with the confirmation I later received with the analysis of my responses to the Myer-Briggs Type Indicator (Myers & Myers, 1995) that intuition, one of the four psychological types heralded by Swiss psychiatrist Carl Jung (1976), figures prominently in my psychological make-up, further emboldened me to embrace my intuitive nature rather than deny it to please those near to me for whom it defied knowing.

Living as a sensing person once again, though, is taking some time. While I welcomed and trusted spontaneous intuitive knowledge, which, for me, often was quite directive, i.e., *"Do this."* Or implicit, i.e., *"She's going to fall."* like the experience of many, as I have learned, including extreme adventurers (e.g., Coffey, 2008), I refrained from seeking it. I trusted I would learn what I needed to do for myself and others as necessary, but I did not want to become generally aware of pain and suffering. I did not want to know, for example, that someone was gravely ill, or desperately unhappy, or suicidal unless I could remove their suffering, which usually engulfed me as I touched it.[3] Naively, I thought it was up to me, Rescuer that I have tended to be (Please see Chapter 2), to remove others' pain and suffering. And I wanted to spare myself the agony I felt when I empathized with their distress. Gradually, I learned through the study of Transactional Analysis and, later, the development of a mindfulness meditation practice that my true responsibility was to remain steady and empathetic with those who were suffering as I compassionately (e.g., Silverman, 2006b) helped them make and implement choices to manage their discomfort. With those understandings in place and by accumulating an increased amount of resources to help those in a variety of circumstances, I became more comfortable living and working as a sensing human being.

Intuitive Communication

The reality of intuitive communication between individuals was poignantly emphasized in a spring, 2007, ABC special television report by Bob Woodruff. Based in part on a memoir he co-authored with his wife Lee (Woodruff and Woodruff, 2007). Mr. Woodruff, former anchor of the ABC evening news, described his ongoing recovery from traumatic head injury caused several months earlier by shrapnel from a roadside attack while on assignment in Iraq. The shrapnel damaged most of his left cerebral hemisphere including the speech and language centers, and he entered a coma. Lee left their children in the care of others to take up residence in the hospital where he was being treated to be with him daily. They said medical staff told her Bob responded differently to her presence than to theirs. Jokingly, he relayed that staff sensed he seemed afraid of her.

On the 38th consecutive day Bob remained in a coma, staff advised Lee to consider nursing home placement for him because he was making physical movements characteristic of those who fail to return to waking consciousness. Alarmed and exhausted from contemplating the consequences of the application of the unwanted recommendation, Lee, late that evening when she was alone, envisioned herself angrily telling Bob to *"Come out of it,"* explaining she had left their children to be with him and that medical personnel were doing everything they could to help him recover, so he needed to do his part and *"Return."* Bob related that he awoke around three a.m. that morning excited to be present. He sat up and waited for Lee to arrive. As she entered the room that morning, he immediately asked, *"What took you so long?"*

We all receive unspoken messages transmitted through the energetic network that supports us all (e.g., Lipton, 2005). Some come in the form of visual images. Some are audible, others are verbal, and some are sensations or emotions. Sometimes we readily recognize the apparent sender. Other times we do not. For instance, one Sunday, many years ago, during a time in my life when I was searching for a faith community to join, I visited a Society of Friends meeting house to sample their communal worship. During silent meditation, I noticed the word *"Theravada"* scrolling letter-by-white letter across the dark inside of my forehead. Technically, the experience was as though watching a special news alert wind across a television screen. I thought I had heard that word. And I thought it was Buddhist. My daughter was majoring in Southeast Asian studies at the time with an emphasis on Buddhist practice and culture. Although she shared very little of what she was learning with me, I thought I had heard her say it. So, as quickly as I could, I returned home to look for *"Theravada"* in the dictionary. I discovered it indeed was a Buddhist word, the name given the original form of Buddhism taught by the Buddha. The practice emphasizes meditation and concentration practices and living a monastic life.

Other intuitive messages may arrive as bodily sensations, feelings, sounds, and, very rarely, smells. For instance, one Saturday morning walking through a shopping mall, I suddenly felt battered, especially in my midsection. I paused and, in a sense of disbelief at the visual image I was receiving of a truck driving straight toward me, said to my companion, *"I feel like I was hit by a truck."* The pain began leaving my body, and we continued shopping. That afternoon, when I returned home, I found a message on my answering machine that my step-mother had been injured in a motor vehicle accident. The car in which she had been a passenger had been hit head-on by a truck at approximately the same time I felt the painful body sensations! Many share this experience of intuitively knowing, or sensing, that someone or something, such as an animal companion who is emotionally close to them, has been hurt or, even, has died (e.g., Williams, 2003). Some messages may arrive during sleep as a dream or part of a dream (e.g., Bosnak, 1985).

Apparently no one reception method is better than another as a clinical tool or a personal guidance system. Noted medical intuitive Caroline Myss (2002a) advises aspiring intuitives to discover and develop their own receptive system. The psychiatrist Judith Orloff (2004), the animal intuitive Marta Williams (2003), and collaborating physicians Mona Lisa Schulz and Christiane Northrup (2005) offer practical guidelines for skillfully practicing and developing intuitive reception. All involve learning to establish a quiet, calm, focused mind and the mindset to attend to what is present each moment, i.e., mindfulness. In addition, personal calibration builds an accurate and reliable resource (e.g., Myss, 2002a).

EMPATHY

Actors do it. So do vocal artists. Successful salespeople rely on it. You do it. And so do I.

What do we do? We show empathy. Actors develop empathy for the characters they portray to depict them honestly. Singers connect with the feelings behind the lyrics to better communicate the meaning of a song. Salespeople reflect our feelings back to us in ways they hope to increase our likelihood of buying their wares. You and I do it when we encounter another who excites our imagination.

We consider empathy as what we come to know after we have walked in another's shoes for a mile. We know it as the ability to understand what another feels and, to some extent, thinks because feelings derive from beliefs. Being empathetic with another does not mean agreeing with that person's point-of-view. It does mean being willing to understand it. Some (e.g., Moore, 2006) think empathy is essential to clinical effectiveness, and I am one. Empathy conveys respect for another's humanness, and without feeling empathy, or knowing, we can not show compassion (e.g., Silverman, 2006b). Compassion, or understanding, expresses itself as the skillful application of empathetic knowledge with the specific intent of relieving suffering, one's own or that of another.

Relieving suffering is what we are about. What other purpose so genuinely satisfies us for doing the work we do? Not to receive awards. Not to garner promotions. Not to earn titles. Not even to receive salary and benefits. We can achieve those benchmarks of successful employment by creating actuarial tables, managing an office, preparing tax returns, or by working in other ways. When we choose to invest our time and dollars earning college degrees that permit us to help people communicate more effectively and to swallow more safely, we do so to relieve their suffering from being misunderstood and from choking from physical complications. That is our primary payoff because, basically, we are empathetic.

But we often need more than a little encouragement to be empathetic with ourselves. Often, we choose to hide our hurt. We do that when we know no other way to cope and want to appear invulnerable. We may think we will cleanse ourselves of the hurt later, but, living the busy lives we do in a culture not easily given to self-reflection and healing, we do not. Instead, we decided often become busier. Eat more, especially more calorie dense, so-called comfort food. Self-medicate with non-nutritional substances to dull the ache or pain we feel. And, then, watch our faces and bodies bulge from the excess weight we drag around and experience unpleasant, derivative somatic sensations from the feel-good substances we ingested. We hurt even more. And we become intensely angry at ourselves and the situations we are creating that only give us more of what we do not want for ourselves or those we care about and for. That is when many of us falsely think being hard on ourselves will help. We berate ourselves for being dumb, which was one of my common self-flagellations, or useless, or, even, hopeless. We become obsessively remorseful. Then, of course, we feel worse. We become increasingly robotic, repeating well-established behavior patterns that allow our thinking mind to dwell on how imperfect we are instead of attending fully to our circumstance and responding appropriately and creatively to what we observe. Being so self-absorbed can lead to clinical depression, even, agoraphobia.

If, instead, we showed ourselves the same empathy, we offer others by recognizing and accepting hurt feelings as inevitable in life and, then, using them as sign posts to learn and problem solve, we would feel strong, even powerful, and, possibly, victorious. Learning to routinely show empathy to ourselves, using kindness, warmth, and patience as buffers, leads to living fulfilling lives, ones in which we can more easily show empathy to others.

Challenges I have found to being effectively empathetic are: 1) Being tempted to offer sympathy when empathy was needed. 2) Thinking that my thoughts and emotions were another's. And 3) Neglecting to responsibly deflect others' excessive emotional demands. I refer to them below respectively as *Us-ness*, *What Is*, and *Guard-All*.

Us-ness

While we prepare a vegetable lasagna, shop for linens, take out the trash, water house-plants, stargaze, walk our dog, day dream, or engage in any other activity of daily life, we silently broadcast our thoughts and feelings. Just as the thoughts and feelings of others come quietly and seemingly unbidden to us, so, too, do our thoughts and feeling arrive at others' personal spaces. Social neuroscientists study this network of unspoken communication (e.g., Goleman, 2006a; 2006b). Among their recent findings are those suggesting we humans are hard-wired for empathy. Daniel Goleman (2006a), for instance, reports that we readily attune to the emotions of others, *if we but attend*. But why should we attend? True, being attuned to members of our families, clans, tribes and villages during ancient times helped create mutually caring, safe communities, in short, helped keep us alive. But, in the 21st century, with our more complicated lifestyles, we rely more on our own wits, including our technological know-how, to support our sense of well-being. For instance, we prize our computers and smart phones that allow us to text, e-mail, and instant message with ease, helping inform us of external threats and providing anxiety-reducing verbal contact with family, friends, work associates, and buddies. We often spend more time relating to each other electronically sharing information than empathetically sharing ourselves.

That may be why so many of us feel isolated. We lack the sense of empathetic immediacy that convinces us we belong. We often feel like a stranger, dog-paddling through a sea of strangers. When we are in the same room as family members, even sitting around the dinner table together, we may be preoccupied with receiving and answering text mail and e-mail and indifferent to the emotions of our partners and children, as they may be to ours, while they, as we, contemplate chatting online or on cell phones with friends to assuage our loneliness.

Our clients demand more. Sr. Anne, for example, referred to in Chapter 1, broke her lengthy silence with rehabilitation staff as a diagnosed "global aphasic" to sternly warn me, *"I need empathy not sympathy!"* I believe she knew before I did that the unspoken sympathy I showered on her was more for my benefit than her own. Identifying this frail, crumpled, presumably linguistically incompetent woman as pitiable allowed me to distance myself from her. That was my shameful strategy as a substitute speech therapist during a brief and awkward co-treatment session with an occupational therapist to relieve myself of the overwhelming sense of ineptness I felt being expected to address her apparent, all-encompassing linguistic needs. I wanted to be seen by that colleague as competent, even more than that, as singularly effective. Successfully meeting any one of Sr. Anne's needs, for which I had had no prior experience, seemed like a possibility so remote as to be improbable. Because I was more concerned with my own welfare than with hers, I only allowed myself to be dimly aware my pity was dismissive. What Sr. Anne seemingly knew was that a therapist viewing her as pitiable interfered with her healing process.

Like conferring a life sentence, offering sympathy can short-circuit growth by reducing expectations for change often to a minimum, since expectations usually become self-fulfilling. At the same time, relating to someone as an object of pity presumes inequality. That act says, *"I am here, and you are there."* Pity separates us by a gulf as infinite an allegorical depiction of the afterlife in which Father Abraham appears across a chasm from sinners. Perceiving a client as pitiable precludes a sense of "us." Without a sense of "Us-ness," the possibility of easing a therapeutic relationship into a partnership encouraging clients to draw fully on their healing resources becomes a remote possibility. Responding empathetically sets the stage for realizing desired change.

What Is

Those trying to explain quantum theory and taking into account the inherent instability of form sometimes insist that the very act of observing prevents the observer from knowing the observed as it is (e.g., H.H. The Dalai Lama, 2005b; Lipton, 2005). They give as a reason: *There is no distinction between what we label as ourselves and what we label as the world outside ourselves.* They assert: *We are the creators of our own reality, both inside and outside of ourselves.*[4] This, perhaps, startling notion is not new. Yogis, Buddhists, Cabbalists, Sufis, and mystics of various traditions have shared this realization for millennia. Even secular psychiatrists, beginning with Sigmund Freud, observed that we have a tendency to subconsciously impute our values, thoughts, and feelings to others, as if our thinking was their own. They call this inclination *projection* (Please See Chapter 1), a tendency writer and diarist Anais Nin wittily described as, *"We do not see things as they are. We see them as we are."* Knowing this puts us on notice to know ourselves!

Clearly, this compelling view of cosmology suggesting all is one coupled with our subconscious tendency to project our thoughts and feelings on those we observe raises quite an obstacle to being empathetic. If we can detect moment-by-moment *whether* we are thinking and *what* we are thinking, we can begin to distinguish our thoughts and feelings from those of the one who interests us. Then, upon reflection, we can say with certainty, *"If I were her, I would be feeling so angry!" "If I were him, I would be so happy."* But, when we witness someone in dire straits, someone with whom we can readily identify, perhaps, a young mother newly diagnosed with an aggressive form of cancer or a doctoral student experiencing memory and cognitive problems following traumatic brain injury from injuries received in a motor vehicle accident, we may quickly and effortlessly project ourselves into the emotional quality of their situation. We become, at least temporarily, unaware of the possible differences between their thoughts and feelings and our own. We believe, *"She should do this." "She should do that." "He should do this." "He should do that."* That is when we need to pull back. We need to refrain from drawing conclusions. We need hold back from giving directives. We need to stabilize. *We need to differentiate.* From the standpoint of quantum mechanics, that may not be theoretically possible until we realize a global shift in consciousness, but behaving as though we can will provide us the best opportunity we have to relate helpfully to each other.

Perhaps, it is clear. Perhaps, it is not. So, let me once again suggest the value of adopting a method to learn to stop, calm, and stabilize the mind. Only by learning to do that, to become well enough acquainted with the working of our own mind can we detect, at any moment whether or not and what we are thinking, can we expect to become effectively empathetic. That being said, since such skillful awareness of the functioning of our mind usually evolves over the long-term, we need to be quite circumspect when we claim to know what another is thinking. While we might be quite correct about sensing what another is feeling, especially if we can see their face, we are less likely to accurately discern *why*, that is what they are thinking that led to the particular feeling or feelings we observe, at least immediately. And, even if we could be absolutely certain we knew what another was thinking, we need to be cautious about how to reveal that we do to avoid suggesting we possess superior powers, even omnipotence, which could invite another to attempt to establish an unhealthy, dependency relationship with us. So, being effectively empathetic requires discernment and tact, and, above all, self-knowledge.

Guard-All

Quite some time ago, transitioning from a career in academia into full-time clinical work with young adults who had incurred traumatic brain injury left me fading fast. The intense emotions I encountered from the patients, members of their support systems, and that of the clinical and support staff drew away more of my energy than I was able to promptly replenish. This was not a new experience for me. All my life, I had been considered sensitive. Although I learned to cope with my sensitivity to circumstances fairly well in an intellectual academic setting, I was on the verge of fatiguing-out after entering this new, emotionally intense environment. The work-day exposure to the intense emotions of fear and anger bouncing off the drywall, the acoustic ceiling tiles, the hard linoleum floors, and each other combined with the draining effects of single-parenting and a participating in a co-dependent relationship was doing heavy damage to my health. I sought help from the popular, charismatic rabbi of the congregation of which I was a member. He seemed to be dealing with many and varied congregants without fading, so I thought he might be willing and able to help me learn to cope with the demands I was facing from the people at work. He agreed to advise me. Expecting to begin a series of classes and maybe some counseling, I was astonished when all he told me was this,

> *"Don't go out without your Guard-All!"*

In case I did not understand this cryptic message, he repeated the advice by chanting the words with an up-beat emphasis. I immediately recognized them as a popular jingle for a brand of toothpaste that had saturated the television airwaves decades earlier. The commercial claimed this toothpaste was different from all the rest. Only this toothpaste protected each tooth. It encased each one in its own cavity-preventing shield, "Guard-All." That's all he said, although he did, from time-to-time, make eye contact with me and quietly chant it anew if he saw me dragging myself around the synagogue.

So, as always, it was up to me to find a solution for a problem of mine and use it. Just as it is, for anyone seeking help. And I did. I concocted Ellen-Marie's refreshing, energy-conserving, all-purpose "Guard-All." I used ingredients culled from writings and recordings, especially those of Carolyn Myss (e.g., 2004a) on personal power use and conservation; Transactional Analysis theory and therapy on setting and maintaining personal boundaries and using cross transactions as *psychological game* stoppers (Berne, 1996); and spiritual practices of various world religions to create a personal cosmology defining giving and receiving. I combined them with a mindfulness meditation practice (e.g., Kornfield, 2001) infused with *shenpa* practice (e.g., Silverman, 2005: Chödrön, 2005b) and Judith Orloff's (2004) suggestions for living healthfully as a sensitive person, including comprehensive tips for successfully dealing with pervasive *energy vampires*, people who, because of deep fear, excessive anger, and/or ignorance, steal others' vital energy to support what they believe they are entitled to have and be. And I stirred in Thich Nhat Hanh's (e.g.,2002) advice to vigilantly guard our sense doors, e.g., our eyes, ears, and mouth, to prevent system contamination from exposure to gratuitous and excessive media presentations of violence and from ingesting mind-altering substances.

How do I use my "Guard-All?" I say, "NO!" --- pure and simple, verbally and non-verbally. I communicate "NO!" to:

- Clients' and caregivers who demand I do their thinking.

- Clients' who expect *me* to cure them while they dare me to try or simply want to see what will happen while I do all or most of the goal-setting and planning.

- Colleagues expecting sympathy when they repeatedly complain about concerns instead of sincerely seeking solutions to the problems that vex them.

- Clients, caregivers, colleagues, students, employees, and anyone, including family, friends, neighbors, and public transportation seatmates, who dramatically demand attention while they talk incessantly draining my energy so they can replenish their own.

I say "NO!" in a timely, confident, and appropriate manner to all who knowingly or unknowingly seek to exploit my knowledge and talent to avoid doing their own work or my gentle, empathetic nature to drain my energy for their own benefit. Consider these scenarios:

Vignette1.

A neighbor runs out of his house within minutes of my beginning work on a gardening task to watch, ask questions, and offer comments drawing my attention and energy away from my work to him. I say, *"Excuse me, but I need to do this work."* Then verbally and physically ignore him. If he continues to try to draw me away from my work, I remove myself from the work area to somewhere less accessible to him or return indoors.

Vignette 2.

A client I have been working with for a while begins a harangue about her roommate, partner, or someone else. I look her in the eye and ask, *"Are you telling me that because you want my help solving your problem?"* Letting her know I am not willing to listen to complaints unless she presents troublesome situations as problems she plans to solve. Incessant complaining (my own as well as others) drains my energy.

Carolyn Myss, medical intuitive (e.g., 1997), claims individuals who chronically complain rather than problem-solve seem to possess tentacle-like structures capable of plugging into others' *third chakra*. The third chakra, or energy center, functions like a storage battery for our personal power. When someone drains it, we feel as though our self-esteem has melted through the floor.

Vignette 3.

A colleague saunters past my cubicle and, sneering, remarks, *"Taking another break?"* I counter her blatant invitation to a *psychological game* (e.g., Berne, 1996) looking directly into her eyes while sincerely posing the counter-query, *"How are you doing today?"*

Someone whose aim is to goad another into anger-motivated speech or behavior does so to create a situation in which they feel dominant. They know angry outbursts weaken others while strengthening their own energetic resources. Countering their invitation to feed them with anger by offering gentle, kind, compassionate responses or silence obviates their intent and encourages them to move on.

Clearly, saying "NO!" is rarely as simple as saying the word, *No*. Saying "NO!" is a total package, i.e., body language, facial expression, vocal tone, and vocal intensity, accompanying a verbal message, which altogether deflects another's invitation to play a harmful psychological game while encouraging a positive exchange and politely and quickly as possible ending an unwelcome one. Effectively saying "NO!" to unwanted intrusions on our attention and energy involves remaining centered and positive. Vigilantly maintaining that stance secures our personal safety zone.

To summarize, donning my permeable, protective "Guard-All" shield deflects unwanted interference with my physical, emotional, and psychic well-being while allowing me to relative positively. And, like the dental "Guard-All," my home brew's protective benefits accumulate with regular use. I grow stronger and healthier each day!

COMPASSION

"Showing compassion to ourselves, we reconcile all beings."

- - - The Tao

My father and stepmother raised my younger sister and me to hate all who differed from them — including myself! Whether it was the single mother living in the house next to ours whose children they thought were poorly dressed and poorly behaved; our tenant in the upstairs flat who benefited from our duplex's poor insulation by enjoying a warmer flat than we did; my wealthy uncle who denied my father's effort to gouge him in a business deal; my mother's parents who satisfied my young child's longing to remember and learn about my mother, who died when I was three and one-half, which my father insisted "poisoned my mind;" or anyone who wittingly or unwittingly defied their expectations of what they thought was right. So, they despised me, the quiet, overly-sensitive, gentle, independent-thinking, bright female child silently grieving the death of her mother, decidedly out-of-place in a household where crudeness, cruelty, and a generalized disdain for strong, educated females held sway.

Superficially, it seems mildly ironic that, as the object of their focused, relentless, decades-long hatred for acting and seeming different, I have chosen to live as compassionately and kindly as possible. Or, perhaps, that is not ironic at all. Those of us who have experienced pervasive suffering in childhood often find it easier to empathize with the suffering of those around us even when the reason for their suffering differs from what we personally have known (Friedman, 2007; Goleman, 2006b). Suffering is suffering. It is pain. It is grief. It is shame. It is desperation. It is longing. It is hurt. It is disillusion. And it can be delusion. Suffering and the desire for relief from suffering is what we all have in common despite differences of age, gender, race, skin color, geography, finances, faith community membership, etc. We can either help relieve the suffering within and around us or add to it. That is one of the most important choices we make individually each day.

Me First

For ill or good, seeking peace and well-being while avoiding pain and hardship drives most of what we say and do, day in and day out and, for some of us, so does the wish to help release others from suffering. In fact, some of us concentrate on relieving other peoples' suffering while neglecting to address our own. We often ignore our needs because we do not want to be considered selfish. We believe Judeo-Christian scripture teaches that caring for oneself is selfish. Inexplicably, we fail to notice that the Golden Rule, *"Love your neighbor as yourself"* (Leviticus 19: 17-19; Mark 12: 28-31), which instructs us to tend to others, contains the words *". . . as yourself"* as a benchmark for how we are to help others. This implies that the standard for our expressions of compassion, i.e., how well we love others, depends on whether and how well we love ourselves. The Golden Rule communicates that self-care is not only primary but righteous. We are no less or no more worthy than others. When we recognize our own suffering and our right to compassionately attend to it, we become more skillful helping identify and relieve the suffering of others. M retelling of an Hasidic tale provides an unexpected, pertinent twist. In brief:

> *Many years ago, in a village in Eastern Europe, a wealthy man chose to live a miserly life. He ate little. He wore tattered clothing. He slept in a hovel and covered himself with rags each evening to protect himself from the cold. And he declined to give money to those who asked.*
>
> *Noticing this, the local rabbi paid him a visit. He advised the man to live in accordance with his means. And, because he knew the rabbi to be wise and compassionate, he followed the rabbi's instructions. He purchased a grand home. He wore elegant clothes. And he dined sumptuously. It was then he understood the meanness of the lives of those who were starving, poorly clothed, and homeless. That was when, as the rabbi surmised, he began showing charity to those who were poor. For the remainder of his life, he gave quietly and unceasingly to others.*

Sometimes we fail to care for ourselves because we feel we do not deserve loving attention and care. My lack of self-worth after years of psychological, emotional, and physical abuse propelled me into a life of doing for others. Not only did I want to relieve others of their suffering, knowing its ill-effects, but I only felt worthwhile when I was engaged in work I thought would benefit others. Working on behalf of others is not bad. But only caring for others is. I neglected my well-being in so many ways. Blessed with a basically sound body from birth but raised among sedentary people at a time when few adults, especially women, regularly exercised, I felt no inclination, as a young adult, to exercise, stretch, rest or to prepare my body well for old age, since I was too blinded to recognize that our bodies unnecessarily deteriorate at an accelerated rate without adequate care and because I did not feel I personally deserved special attention. Now I am paying quite an unnecessary price in limited mobility, and I am giving my physical body all the loving attention I can.

With kindness toward ourselves, we can skillfully put empathy into action not only for ourselves but also for others applying kindness and warmth. And that is compassion (Silverman, 2006b). If no one has taught us to be kind to ourselves, then that is something we can do for ourselves and, ultimately, for others. In the main, that means learning to understand.

5   RIGHT AND WRONG I: WHAT IS

"In each life, there are 10,000 joys and 10,000 sorrows."

- - - *The Buddha*

Arising in the morning, we commonly attend to our body and mind to see what's going on with us. We quickly notice any stiffness, pain, bloating, or other atypical sensation. We also notice any anxiety, dread, anger, impatience we may be feeling. But we rarely notice how well we are doing: We rise, make it to the bathroom, empty our bladder and, perhaps, evacuate our bowels, notice the birds singing and chattering while we wash and brush our teeth, say *"Love, ya!"* to our precious other stretching out on our bed, dive into our closet to find something suitable to wear, and off we go. We are doing quite well.

We have a new day to learn and do. We have the opportunity to help each other and our planet become better. But few of us adopt this outlook. Instead, we only seem to concern ourselves with how to manage everything and everyone around us to keep our lives from going wrong. How dreary! But, more than that, how awful!

No wonder so many of us feel weighted down, heavy, leaden, and joyless. When we narrow our outlook to only notice what is wrong with us, each other, our city, village, country, planet, and universe, and when we only focus on what we must do to keep our life from unraveling, we become stupefied. How good it feels when, occasionally, someone catches our eye as we stand in the checkout lane at the market and gives us a bright, warm smile, as if to say, *"It's all right, Sister. Life is bigger and better than this!"* and we smile back the same 100-watt smile, acknowledging we do know that is true: Life is bigger and better than our impatience at waiting in line. And, for the few minutes immediately thereafter, while we savor the feel of the smile we received and the smile we sent radiating through our body and energizing it, we feel light and lighter. We feel hopeful. We feel connected with a positive pulse that convinces us we matter, and we are doing fine. Then, as we allow our thoughts to snap back to our concerns about being late for dinner, getting to the theater on time afterward, finishing the laundry after we return home, gassing up the car tomorrow morning as we begin our commute to the city, the light behind our eyes dims, our limbs feel heavy once more, and we feel exhausted and sad. We begin thinking, once again, that our life is meaningless, just a series of endless tasks interspersed with pangs of anxiety. Our spine imperceptibly crumples. Our eyes see less and less. Our ears take a break as we listen primarily to our own thoughts and concerns. We're back in our dimly lit bubble, feeling oppressed and discouraged. This is a really grim depiction of daily life. But not so different from what most of us experience. We are like riders on run-away horses which drag us here, there, and wherever they wish to go, and we either go along for an anxious ride of indeterminate length, pull-back smartly on the reins, saying *"Whoa!!"* until she stops, or fall off.

The run-away horse is a metaphor for our thoughts often arising from anger, fear, and doubt. When we occupy ourselves with these energies, we easily can spin out an incredible volume of compelling and disturbing thoughts. For instance,

❖ *"Will I raise my GPA in time to be a serious candidate for graduate school?"*

> May lead to:

>> *Should I drop some of my courses to raise my GPA?*

>> *Should I add some courses to raise my GPA?*

>> *Should I explain I had to work 20 hours a week?*

>> *I wonder if strong recommendations will offset my GPA*

>> *or maybe a strong GRE score . . .*

>> *Maybe if I took off a year to work as a speech assistant . . .*

>>> *Etc.*

>>> *etc.*

>>> *etc.*

❖ *"How long will it take for me to pay off all these student loans?"*

> May lead to:

>> *I'm not going to be able to live the way I want or save much money while I'm paying back those loans.*

>> *I should see a loan officer to learn how long I'll be paying for them.*

>> *I wish my Dad had leant me the money, but he's never done anything for me.*

>> *None of my friends have to worry about paying off student loans.*

>>> *Etc.*

>>> *etc.*

>>> *etc.*

❖   *"How can I be sure putting off marriage until I'm 30 will be what I want?"*

    May lead to:

        I won't be happy being married if I don't travel as I planned.

        I'm too unsettled to commit to a life-time relationship.

        What if he finds someone else before I'm ready to marry?

        What if I become too set in my ways by the time I'm 30 to

        enjoy the healthy give-and-take of a committed relationship?

            Etc

                etc.

                    etc.

    And

❖   *"Moving out-of-state seems like a good idea, but how do I know I'll be able to find friends and enjoy life as much as I do here?"*

    May lead to:

        I've never been good at making new friends.

        It will take a while to develop a support network in a new place.

        Things aren't so bad here.

        I could move from my parents' home into a near-by

        apartment to try living on my own.

            Etc.

                etc.

                    etc.

And so it goes. Each primary thought can lead to a barrage of related ones that can occupy our attention day and night, often increasing our anxiety as we mull over unknowns. Life around us becomes nothing but a blur as it does to riders of run-away horses. We fail to notice the warmth of the sun on our face and back, the coolness of the air as we slice through it while power-walking at sunrise, the fragrance of the lilac blossoms filling the moisture laden air, and the geese honking overhead as they wend their way south in a five body v-formation. Speeding along on a seemingly chaotic journey, we feel only mounting anxiety. *Where are we headed? Will we arrive safely? Will we be happy there?* We see only what is wrong or what may go wrong. We feel no joy and have none to share. It is time to stop the horse and dismount. We need to take another look at what is, and we know how.

Pentimento

Award winning playwright and author Lillian Hellman published a three-volume autobiographical memoir entitling the second volume *Pentimento* (Hellman, 2000), a term borrowed from curators and art historians to identify artists' modifications of all or part of a completed painting. She wanted to look anew at certain events and people who shaped her life to see whether they exerted the influence she once thought. A sensitive, mature woman she had learned life is more richly dense than it first may seem. She knew that, given a different perspective, an alternate conclusion may better fit the interpretation of an observation or circumstance made earlier. An ubiquitous, streamlined example of what she intended is interpreting the meaning of a goblet filled to 50% capacity. Upon viewing, some consider it half-full, others half-empty. These divergent conclusions highlight the subjective quality of conclusions drawn about a seemingly objective circumstance. What we consider favorable differs from what we consider unfavorable primarily by elements that shape our perception, not the object of perception itself. And these influential elements, at the deepest level, happen to be our *core beliefs*. For instance, if I believed *No Good Ever Comes To Me*, I probably would conclude such a goblet to be half-empty because that belief predisposes me to consider whatever I encounter to be flawed in some way. But if, to the contrary, I believed *Only Good Comes to Me*, I probably would consider that very same goblet half-full because I expect fullness in life. And so it is that challenging our beliefs, which give rise to our thoughts, judgments, and conclusions about ourselves, others, and the world around us, as Hellman did, to see what is actually there brings greater clarity to our relationships and to our life (e.g., Katie, 2003; 20007; Silverman, 2006c).

Spending personal time quietly reflecting upon our behavior to uncover core beliefs, rather than talking about our experiences with friends and others, brings insight required for desirable growth. By contrast, casual talking about our satisfying or perplexing experiences generally serves motives other than stimulating deep personal change. Talking can help relieve the anxiety we feel when alone (e.g., Myss, 2002c) and draw closer those we wish to be intimates. But such ego-driven behavior can get us into jams sooner or later when those to whom we have interacted feel used as ego-supports rather than appreciated as confidantes. On the other hand, quietly centering ourselves as a basis for detecting our core beliefs can only help. When reflective, we come to see dimensions of ourselves and circumstances more clearly to appreciate the fullness of our being (e.g., Kabat-Zinn, 2005).

When we choose to spend more time experiencing life than thinking and talking about it, we discover that only by experiencing life do we actually live it.

WHAT IS RIGHT

More Than We Customarily Acknowledge

One of the daily prayers recited after the morning toilet in the Jewish tradition is an expression of gratitude for the healthy functioning of the body's many ducts and glands, something we, otherwise, might take for granted because, after all, we are referring to the production and elimination of urine and feces. Teaching us to be thankful our bodies remove waste provides a wake-up call. Our bodies do so much for us, and we usually take what they do for granted. We rarely take the time to appreciate our eyes, which bring us wondrous sights to ponder and information about our welfare and the welfare of others; our ears, which allow us to experience the wonderful world of music and to hear each other and the sounds of life around us; our taste buds, which can make eating a delightful experience; our nose, which responds to fragrances and odors that surround and inform us moment-by-moment; our heart, venous system, limbs, muscles, joints, sinews, and skin, which keep us alive, protected, and mobile. Unless we detect a malfunction, we ignore the various parts and systems of our body. Then we become anxious. We wonder what *that* means. We wonder whether our lives will change and how. We can become obsessed with what we are and might be losing. We fail to appreciate all that is right with us each and every moment. There is so much right about our bodies, our values, our intentions, and the physical support system we have acquired, e.g., our homes, cars, yards, wardrobes, friends, families, bank accounts, jobs, hobbies, etc., that we take for granted. If one of the tires on our car goes flat, how wonderful we feel when we resume driving after changing it. We feel so fortunate having a car that runs to give us so much freedom. As we recover from the flu and become able to sip water and eat a bit of toast, we feel we are so lucky to drink and eat again. How we savor the coolness of the water sliding down our throats, pooling in our stomach. How we enjoy the aroma and taste of warm, whole wheat toast and appreciate the act of chewing once again. How we rejoice in the return of our physical strength and mental focus as our body assimilates these gifts of food and drink. These are daily gifts we, otherwise, fail to notice. *Imagine how much different we, as well as clients and caregivers, would feel each day if we consciously appreciated all that is right with us.*

Expressions of Gratitude

We direct so much of our attention to what is wrong, we sometimes fail to notice that so much is right. Keeping a *gratitude journal* helped me restore that balance in my life. Identifying then writing about one experience daily that unexpectedly reminded me life is beautiful brings many more smiles to share. The film "Life is Beautiful (1998)," which received an Academy Award in 1998 for Best Foreign Language Film, depicts how believing life is rich and full can make our lives bearable during even the most challenging times. But most of us, most of the time, do not need to fantasize that life is beautiful. We only need to attend. When we observe a flower in bloom, listen to Mahler's 9th symphony, smell coffee brewing as we arise on a bright Sunday morning, or receive the unsolicited affection of our dog, we know life is good. And, on a basic level, recognizing we have suitable shelter, healthy and sufficient food, adequate clothing, the ability to care for ourselves, available transportation, and freedom to express ourselves and go where we might reminds us we are well-off, a reality obscured by much of media presentations of daily life. We do face challenges individually and collectively, often daily, but we also have resources to draw upon at those times, including our personal strength.

Focusing on what is right, not as a naïve, ineffective Pollyanna, but as a matter of perception, draws in life. We become nourished by associating with what we consider desirable and depleted by what we believe to be destructive (e.g., Orloff, 1996). Limiting time spent listening to or reading the daily news, which we all know is primarily an account of the worst happenings of the day, and time spent with those who seek to fault-find and complain rather than encourage keeps us fresher than we would become if we became slimed by all that destructive content. Familiarizing ourselves with constructive activities in our neighborhoods and towns, in our nation, and around the globe raises our spirits and vitality. How good when we remember ". . . *it's not all about me."* (Mipham, 2007) and then help one another. *And how good our clients, too, can feel when we, by our attitude and action, help inform them there is so much right with them and teach them how to capitalize on their strengths.*

WHAT IS WRONG

We're Not the Only One

Every now and then, we encounter a difficult patch, maybe several. That is when we can become ensnared by faulty thinking such as believing that our whole life is troubled. That sort of distortion can be accentuated by also believing we're the only one who has trouble, or this particular problem. My father suffered from these companion delusions. True, he had his share of problems, some very major ones, in fact. His first wife died of cancer leaving him with two sons, aged eight and 14. Within a few years, he married my mother who died when I was three and one-half within two weeks of delivering my sister by C-section. Seven years later, the older of his two sons, developed testicular cancer and died at the age of 23. That was when he began moaning almost daily, *"Why does everything bad happen to me?"* and *"Why do I have such bad luck?"* whenever he encountered even more ordinary challenges. And, when life seemed flat, he manufactured problems for himself and others by initiating feuds with relatives because he had become emotionally dependent on feeling beleaguered. He seemed incapable of appreciating and enjoying every day life. As far as I know, he took the false belief to his grave that no one was more unlucky than he.

An Invitation to Learn

There are those who believe that what we consider going wrong in our lives actually can be something going right. I am one (e.g., Silverman, 2007b), and here is one reason why:

> *Just last week, my laptop computer malfunctioned by slowing down, then freezing after a hard boot. The PC crawled from page-to-page as I surfed the internet, then seemed clogged and, finally, became unresponsive when I tried to sign off. After trying various remedies that failed to solve this increasingly annoying and frightful problem, I took it to the dealer for diagnosis and repair. Later that same day, I called the repair shop to find out whether I needed to replace the hard drive, which I was fairly certain was breaking down. I was stunned to hear the tech describe the laptop as working "perfectly." He, with a slight smile in his voice, advised me that I needed to let it ". . . do it's own thing," which meant allowing it the time it needed to move from action to action.*
>
> *With only the slightest bit of self-reflection, I recognizedthat my long-standing desire to have what I wanted when I wanted it had forced the problem. Realizing that, I immediately became grateful for the interruption to my life and work caused by the laptop's malfunctioning despite the anxiety, lengthy drive time, and service charges involved to set it right. What I learned about myself by sorting through the problem was worth all that: The source of the problem was within me! While the laptop was busy trying to respond to a request I made, I, impatiently, made another and, sometimes, even another, over-loading its hapless processor. That was me all right! I seek instantaneous responses to my often multiple requests and queries, then become frustrated when I seem to receive no response at all. This was the most obvious message I had yet received that I needed to practice due consideration. I interpreted it as the Universe putting me on notice. I decided to practice patience by learning to live with realistic lag-times with others and with other things trying to respond to my perceived needs and to start by letting my laptop "Do its own thing."*

I have had so many experiences where I learned by looking inward when something in my life seemed to go wrong that it was time for me to change how I was thinking and acting that I have come to consider these initially annoying events as wake-up calls to claim a more expansive life.

Others think this way, too (e.g., Chödrön, 2007). But I realize there are many, like my father, who chose to view such happenings as hurtful instead of helpful to justify their belief, *"No one is more unlucky than I."* and to proclaim loudly that is so in the hope of drawing sympathetic attention to their plight. In fact, I, myself, have done that from time-to-time only to learn that the net result was to live a form of painful, growth-denying, suspended animation, i.e., residing in the *"Poor Me Cocoon!"*

Of course, there are those who satisfy themselves with mechanistic explanations for the appearance of unexpected events, e.g.,

- *There must be an electrical short in the car for the battery to need such frequent replacement.*

- *Lightening struck the house because it is the tallest structure in the area.*

- *The pipes burst because the water pressure was too high for the joints.*

These only superficially satisfy the key question, *"Why?"* That is why I believe expecting behavioral science research results based on group statistical designs to completely satisfy our desire to understand those who seek our assistance is a belief misplaced (Silverman, 2003b; 2003c).[1] At best, such an approach can provide only a glimpse into conditions and circumstances of interest, intellectually satisfying as those tidbits may be. We long for theories that offer sweeping vistas of human life and experience. Viewing events and situations that seem to go wrong as spiritually-inspired challenges to awaken to the deep complexity of life and the value of assuming personal responsibility have given me an outlook that has led to greater professional satisfaction and more personal happiness than my pity-seeking father experienced. Life's speed bumps do that when we let them.

We all know of inspirational individuals, such as Stephen Hawking, the theoretical physicist, living and working with ALS; the late actor Christopher Reed, who, after suffering a spinal cord injury, benefited untold other individuals with spinal cord injuries; and the innumerable people, who devote their lives to creating opportunities for others as a testament to the lives of loved ones they lost. These people help us recognize that personal attitudes determine our satisfaction with life despite physical barriers to living as others. Pain and disappointment can be a very good teachers (Silverman, 2007b) if they encourage us to look within as well as without ourselves to find meaning, sustenance, and guidance.

There are those of us who seem to require high challenges to motivate us to do our best daily and to appreciate the gift of life. Not just mountain climbers or record-setting victors of other extreme challenges but individuals like you and me, who quietly build businesses, begin charitable organizations, invent products that enhance the quality of life, and live a life of service who, respond to the challenge of "no pain, no gain." Again and again, in the process of working to achieve our dreams, we meet disappointment, even adversity. But we bounce back. There is a saying among Hasidic Jews that the *tzadik*, a righteous person who lives by faith, falls seven times and rises seven times. Similarly, Thomas Edison proclaimed, after yet another apparent failure as he sought to invent the incandescent electric light bulb, *"I haven't failed. I just found another way that won't work!"* And on he went. And on we go. We realize learning what does not seem to help us go where we wish teaches us what not to do. Those who seek more learn more and realize failure is a form of success.

Clients who think similarly successfully negotiate the inevitable experience of *relapse*. When they occasionally revert to an unwanted manner of thinking and acting that was once habitual while in the process of learning new, desired patterns, they, with animosity toward none, especially themselves, resume applying the new strategies and practices they prefer. In this way, relapse can help lead to success by strengthening our awareness that what we do is up to us.

Most of us simply prefer "no pain." We value the comfort and security of routine. We attempt to manage change so we face as little disruption as possible to what we like about our lives. The challenge of facing the unknown with all our intelligence and all our strength is not as exciting to us as living predictably, i.e., knowing who we will walk with in the morning, where we will shop for groceries, which schools our children will attend, etc. We crave security. That is why we cling to employment we do not want primarily to secure a desirable retirement package, refuse promotions that remove us from our comfortable departmental *niche*, sing songs of praise to department heads encouraging them to remain just as they are so we can continue to experience what we have known, and so on. And so it is with many of the clients and caregivers we encounter, who, after all, are no less human than we and, like we, will not change until they are willing to take on the new and uncertain.

WHAT ABOUT THERAPY?

What we think is wrong can be right. And what we think is right can be wrong. Those statements may sound like chatter among guests at the Mad Hatter's tea party, or possibly song lyrics , but, actually each can be on the mark, although we can not always be sure how in the moment. It may take some time to discover whether a certain event has helped or hindered us in finding our way and living it, as hindsight often shows. But what we do know is this: *Focusing on what we think is wrong leads us to notice more of what we think is wrong, just as focusing on what we presume to be right draws our attention to more of what we consider right.* That is a result, in part, of an *a priori* belief influencing our perception of reality (e.g., Korbzybski, 1955), which is the basis for what we know as *self-fulfilling prophesy.* That may be why Albert Einstein reportedly said that the most important decision we need to make for ourselves is whether we live in a friendly universe that supplies all our needs or one that requires endless struggle to survive. For instance, if I expect today to go badly because I believe my Mondays always do, I will scan for evidence throughout the day that all is not going right for me. I will notice and focus on: The several red lights I encountered traveling from one work site to another; my difficult to negotiate, fractured work schedule because of many new patient admissions; the loss of my lunch break because I needed to meet with clients instead, and so on. That evening, I could easily conclude as I zoned-out in front of the T.V. mindlessly eating my way across my dinner plate that I had an awful work day as I recounted those frustrating events. To reach that conclusion, I would need to ignore or down-play the fact that one client was able to manage a diet up-grade, another was consistently using short sentences to answer questions rather than one-word responses and gestures, the student therapist showed increasing insight and creativity conducting her sessions, and my car started on the first turn of the key in the ignition despite sitting in 20° below zero wind chill temperatures for five hours.

That mirrors what I did when I steadfastly believed *"The day will go wrong."* It's not simply that expecting the worst brings the worst but that expecting the worst causes us to look for the worst and overlook the rest. That is why some believe therapy focusing on what is wrong with clients abridges their lives by screening from view that which would allow them to experience richer, fuller lives (e.g., Hahn, 2004; Myss, 2002), and I agree.

Balance

Consider for a moment how you might feel about yourself if a therapist unexpectedly approached you and said, *"You don't walk right. You should be in therapy to correct that."* If you had no awareness or concern about how you walked, you might refuse to believe what she told you, but you might not be able to dismiss the thought that there was something wrong with how you walked, indeed, that there was something wrong with you, because, after all, she is an expert. That very thought might make you unusually self-conscious as you went about your daily life. Instead of concentrating on your friend, the scenery, and the people and animals all around as you walked through the neighborhood after dinner, you might study how you were walking to discover what was wrong with you. Such self-conscious attention to how you walked might even cause you to falter now and then, even stumble and trip. Noticing that, you might begin to believe there really was something wrong with you. And like many in this society, you might think more about what was wrong with you and what that might mean than what was right. You might begin to close down.

Now, suppose the "you" that received that judgment from a therapist was not you as an adult but you as a five-year-old. Don't you think your self-concept would be put into jeopardy by an expert introducing doubt about your ability to fit in? Don't you think such doubt would lead you to experience a certain anxiety about whether you were "good enough" or ever would be "good enough?" Of course, there are many factors at play in this hypothetical *scenario*, for example, how self-confident you were before you received this unexpected news, how believable you found adults' opinions, how well you communicated your concerns with your parents, and how satisfactorily they helped you deal with them before the therapist spoke with you, and so on. But if you, as a five-year-old, were like one of the many who care about what others thought of you because you did not want to be abandoned or excluded and vulnerable, you might begin to fear you might not fit in. While we, as adults, might reach a very different conclusion, a child with limited knowledge and experience, a less mature cognitive apparatus, and caregivers possibly ill-equipped to help them deal well with their feelings ordinarily would not.

Just yesterday, I received a call from a father searching for help for his young adult son, who apparently has great difficulty speaking. A colleague alerted me I might since she had suggested they contact me, but, even with that advance warning, I was quite unprepared for what Sam, the caller, told me.

> *With slow precisely articulated speech and a monotone voice oozing despair and deep anger, he recited a series of statements to inform me of what was wrong with Ethan, his son, after he introduced himself, and I inquired how I might be of help. According to Sam, he and his wife were informed by public school personnel when Ethan was five that he had speech and language problems and a learning disability. The school district provided therapy for Ethan until he began high school. That was when the school district encouraged their students to decide whether or not they wanted to continue treatment. Ethan opted out of therapy. Currently, a recent high school graduate, Ethan does landscape work, and according to Sam, is experiencing more difficulty communicating than ever. He enumerated:*
>
> *Ethan has 'no expressive language whatsoever.' He doesn't form sentences because of his limited vocabulary. He stutters more often and more severely than ever, i.e., blocking then trying to force his way through the block. When that fails, he spells the word he stuttered. In restaurants, he scans the menu to identify items he thinks he can say and orders those rather than the ones he actually wants. He does not use the phone.*
>
> *Then, having completed the list of what was wrong with Ethan, he relaxed and, breathing more deeply and employing animated speech and vocal characteristics, proudly added that Ethan had been active in high school sports and hung out with a group of guys whose friendship he maintains.*

Until that final disclosure, I was concerned Sam only seemed to image Ethan as someone whose life was going dismally wrong and even may be irredeemable. But the pride and caring evident in that final comment led me to realize Sam also saw at least some of what was right with Ethan. Without the awareness that things were right with Ethan as well as wrong, he could cripple Ethan. With it, he could help him draw on his strengths to live as well as he might.

Starting With Ourselves

Starting with ourselves, we learn to notice and appreciate that even when we are sad and disappointed we can experience moments of peace, joy, and calm. We can notice the leafing out of our silver maple, a robin resting in our Hawthorne tree the first time this spring, the culinary skills of our teen-age daughter, the skilled welding skills of our 17 year-old son, the arching of trees across our city street, and so on. These moments refresh us, infuse us with life. They encourage us to live with appreciation and reverence. These moments are needed more than ever when we are disappointed and dissatisfied with ourselves. They steady us, center us. They help us draw from all that is enduring. They provide the necessary mix that is wholesome life. To focus on what saddens us to the exclusion of recognizing joyful experiences deprives us of life-giving support. It weakens us. That can be the downside of therapy that focuses on what is wrong with clients.

So often when we focus change on our problems and what we are doing wrong, *we think we need to eliminate what is wrong to make ourselves right.* That reasoning is a little like convincing ourselves we need to go to war to have peace when what we need to do is to grow the peace within our own hearts until love and compassion inform all we think and do. The consequence of focusing on what is wrong with ourselves to make ourselves right is that we may begin to think and act as though we are flawed. We may begin to believe we can't do things right. Our spirit plummets. We loose self-esteem. We may even loose interest in life. True, clients may approach therapy with these dark thoughts and feelings, e.g., the 10-year old main character in *Jason's Secret*, (Silverman, 2001), but therapy that focuses on what is wrong with clients magnifies those unhealthy beliefs. This attitude overlooks the stark reality that we are fine just as we are (e.g., Berne, 1996). *All we need to do is to learn to do something different than we have done before.*

A certain awareness of what we are doing wrong remains an essential ingredient of successful therapy. After all, we do not wish to continue thinking and behaving in ways we find counter-productive. We want to do something else. We want to get somewhere else. Of course, some of us wish we could just *be* someone else, someone more fluent, someone with a more authoritative voice, someone who could remember appointments without having to write them all down, etc. or be somewhere where people were friendlier, life was lived at a slower pace, etc. We are not always so eager to do the work required to become as we wish (e.g., Silverman, 2007a). But, with thought and imagination, we can readily find ways to cultivate behaviors that allow us to act as we wish for as long as we use them. For instance, we can monitor our breathing so that we speak on the outbreath rather than holding our breath as we speak the way we do when we try to avoid stuttering. Noticing that holding our breath to avoid stuttering intensifies our stuttering problem, we decide to approach speaking differently. Of course, we can avoid holding our breath when we speak. But that avoidance behavior stresses us as we struggle to succeed. On the other hand, we can decided to speak on the outbreath and practice doing so, first on small speech units then larger and larger ones culminating with conversation. We discover focusing on what to do rather on what not to do we become more successful because we eliminate much of the cause of unhealthy stress that derives from an avoidance orientation. Similarly, we can speak with a wider mouth opening rather than clenching our jaw when we speak to increase the volume of our voice without stressing the respiratory to produce greater and more expiratory effort. And, we can keep an appointment book rather than relying exclusively on our memory. And as long as we continue doing what helps us accomplish what we wish, we will accomplish what we wish.

Another reason to concentrate on cultivating desirable behaviors rather than on suppressing unwanted ones is that we all have a tendency to identify ourselves with our behavior. For instance, when we care for our garden and witness it produce healing herbs, fresh, tender vegetables, luscious fruit, and vibrant flowers, we often feel generous, giving, and accomplished. When we fail to water and weed it allowing it to shrivel and fail, we may feel derelict, even worthless. Similarly, if we speak in public despite the possibility we may stutter rather than stifling our thoughts, we may feel strong, perhaps, masterful even if we stutter in the process. But, if we shun the opportunity to talk to others, we can feel pinched and useless. That is how clinical strategies that lead clients to identify with their strengths and help cultivate new ones not only can result in meeting personal goals but can establish a wholesome learning environment in general. For instance, if we wish to become kinder and more compassionate, we can do so by deciding to perform one act of kindness daily. Most of us already know how to be kind, and we know how to be compassionate. What we need to accomplish is to act kindly and compassionately more often. As we begin to behave kindly and compassionately once each day, we may soon discover we are spontaneously performing multiple acts of kindness and compassion daily because we enjoy the warmth and expansiveness of spirit we feel when we do. We even may find that our thoughts about ourselves and others are becoming more compassionate and less judgmental regardless of whether or not we act on them. If we had focused on being less mean, perhaps, less selfish, we would be far less likely to become more kind and compassionate. Chances are the only change we probably would experience would be to become more critical, which, in a sense, is more mean.

And, if we do not know how to be kind, we can start by learning how to be generous. Each day we can place a prized possession in one hand and then transfer it to the other. As we learn to release it from one hand to give it to the other, we can then learn to release other things within our metaphorical grasp to give them to others, and, in the process of giving to others, we will find that being kind involves the doing of which we are capable, i.e., giving what we value to others. *We can extend the lessons from this example to learn to communicate more effectively for the benefit of others as well as ourselves.*

Drawing on Strengths to Fashion New Skills

Consider, for a moment, the historical approaches to stuttering therapy. Traditionally, there have been two different objectives: One has been to focus on increasing fluency. The other has concentrated on eliminating stuttering. While it may seem they are identical since increasing fluency would necessarily reduce stuttering and decreasing stuttering would invariably increase fluency, a selection of focus is essential. In my experience, helping clients apply skills they demonstrate most of the time they talk to modify their occasional stuttering and to envision themselves as people who can talk to anyone at any time even though they may sometimes stutter brings more satisfying change than strengthening clients' misperception that they need to rid themselves of stuttering in order to fit in or have a chance of doing so. After all, such self-denigration creates much of what we consider stuttering problems to be. We do not provide help to those who already practice such thinking and behavior by asking them to do more of the same.

When I was an undergraduate majoring in speech correction, as the profession was labeled then, I became captivated by the concepts introduced in a film shown in an education class. The film featured the belief and practices of a female child psychologist who had been educated and trained in Germany or Austria, based on her accent. Unfortunately, I do not remember her name. She tested children to discover what was right with them! She searched for their strengths, then encouraged teachers and other caregivers to build on these strengths as they taught them new skills. Her approach radically contrasted with what I had been learning in other classes and from studying faculty and students working at the university speech clinic.

Clinicians in the clinic focused on correcting what they thought was wrong with the way clients spoke, usually education majors who had failed speech screening tests and were required to successfully complete speech therapy to receive their degree. Quite often, these clinicians spent several introductory sessions trying to convince the skeptical and, often, antagonistic clients they how they failed to speak properly. They also applied this approach to children with articulation errors and clients of varying ages and communication challenges. In fact, this approach constituted the matrix of therapy in all venues I have come to know, i.e., preschool, middle school, high school, inpatient rehabilitation, outpatient rehabilitation, skilled nursing facility, and home health where the approach had been to transform clients from doing things wrong or not at all into doing things right (e.g., Silverman, 2003b). I, on the other hand, have taken the approach suggested by the European child psychologist to discover individuals' strengths and then to associate them with the goals they wish to meet by building on those strengths to meet personal communication and swallowing needs. Beginning with and building upon success, I witnessed many clients accomplish more than I would have predicted and increase their self-concept significantly in the process.

I recall Susan, a young woman with traumatic brain injury, who, when she first became my client, was angry to the point of being defiant, partly because her previous speech pathologist consistently reminded her of what she did that was incorrect. I reminded her of what she was already doing satisfactorily. We shaped those strengths into new articulatory and cognitive skills to help her meet her goals of wanting to speak clearly enough to ask for information and engage in conversation without being asked *"What?"* after each utterance and of making and following daily schedules for herself. After she and I had been working together for several months, the department supervisor returned from pregnancy leave. Upon seeing this client for the first time since she had left, she literally gasped. She took me aside and gushed, *"She doesn't look like the same person."* Susan had gone from being sullen and untidy to friendly and well put together because she had been slowly, but consistently learning to speak more clearly and plan her daily schedule more effectively and felt successful once again.

Since most of us come to therapy because we want to change something about ourselves or because someone who cares for us thinks we should, this seems entirely reasonable at first, at least on the surface. But, by addressing what is wrong with us and ignoring or down-playing what is right, the net effect of the therapy experience can be demoralizing for all involved. Imagine the cumulative effect on someone's self-concept who had been convinced to enroll in therapy to remediate a problem therapists insisted kept them from being accepted and then not changing appreciably after months or even years of therapy all the while being chastised that what they were doing was wrong.. This possibility needs to be considered well by all of us who attempt to enroll a potential client oblivious and unconcerned about being different. Can we be certain that if we convince an individual to engage in therapy with us to change we will be able to help them reach the goals we have stated they need to meet? If not, we need to forgo such an approach, which is often how we initiate therapy with children.

Beginning by identifying clients' strengths that can be shaped to into skills to help them reach individual goals stimulates a positive attitude. That seems to have been the primary goal of articulation deep-testing, for example, which uses pictures or sentences to stimulate phone production in singletons and blends to identify phonemic environments where a phone customarily misarticulated is produced acceptably. Building on those existing successes became the starting point of therapy, if needed. When, for example, we help clients identify words containing /s/ which they produce without their customary lisp and demonstrate to clients who have stuttering problems they can speak fluently at times during choral reading, we may help raise their self-esteem and jump-start a successful program of therapy.

In contrast, many of the clients I knew in an outpatient rehabilitation program for young adults with traumatic brain injury felt inadequate as a side-effect of their enrollment in the program. Facing the reality of their situation was seen as a necessary aspect of recovery. Because of cognitive deficits, many did not fully appreciate the extent of their memory and reasoning impairments that could jeopardize their own and others' well-being so it was necessary to alert them to such reality. But, failing to also highlight their existing strengths generated an unbalanced sense of self, resulting in unnecessary pessimism. For instance, one day, upon entering the therapy room we used, a client glanced at the anatomical bust of the right half of an adult head and neck sitting on a credenza and said, with only the slightest suggestion of humor, *"That's me. Half-A-Brain."* Until then I had not realized that even he, who seemed so aloof saw himself as decidedly limited. When we see ourselves as limited, we are.

Creating experiences for clients to help them recognize they are useful members of society even as they need help boosts their commitment to change. I noticed young adults with traumatic brain injury often felt useless because staff expectations did not include the possibility that these individuals might give as well as receive advice, information, and encouragement. The prevailing belief seemed to be that the clients' role was exclusively that of consumer of the services offered them. In a society, where what we do helps establish our sense of self-worth, these individuals, most of whom were male, found themselves saddled with the professional staff's expectation that they were to assume a passive, or receptive role in therapy. The implicit attribution by staff of them as non-contributors made a strong statement, which they may have interpreted to imply that also would be their role in life from then on. Surmising that, I created experiences, such as group caroling on Christmas Eve Day, and group therapies where these individuals could visibly contribute to the welfare of group members as they addressed their own speech, language, memory, cognitive, and/or swallowing goals. In those circumstances, they seemed more buoyant and alive than in other activities in the facility where their role was "Recipient of Services." Not that, in their free time, they disregarded one another. Several, in fact, developed close, caring, give-and-take relationships with one another as they spent five days per week for several months at the facility. But the staff, whose opinions carried great weight, positive or negative, fairly uniformly failed to partner with these clients, implying they had little to offer even to themselves.

Many years later, I heard it said, *"If you want to be happy, think of others. If you want to be miserable think of yourself."* I have never read or heard it said that clients happy because they feel useful are more likely to succeed than discouraged ones, but I believe it is so.

Therapy that recognizes and balances what is right with us with what is wrong with us and stems from a practical, outlook is therapy that can provide the help needed.

Beliefs As Architects

Our beliefs serve as the architects of our everyday worlds. That may be why Albert Einstein insisted the most important decision we need to make for ourselves is whether we believe the world to be a supportive presence or an adversarial one because, once we decide, that is what we will live. But we need to cut ourselves some slack. All is not what it first seems (e.g., Hellman, 2000). If we rush to judgment, we may create unnecessarily challenging circumstances for ourselves and others.

As the adage suggests, *Marry in haste; repent at leisure.*   Hastily choosing to believe clients are flawed as opposed to believing they are people with strengths needing development, like everyone else, engenders significant consequences for us and those we serve. It is so easy for us to do. We are, after all, trained as clinicians to notice deviations from the ordinary in people's thinking, emotions, and behavior not their strengths as people and as learners. Once we decide someone performs differently from others of their gender and age who share linguistic, cultural, and educational backgrounds, we only need to make one small step to conclude he or she *is* different. Then we may conclude this individual needs our services to help them fit in. Relatedly, we believe we must show the way and that it is we who must decide what experiences and in what sequence to offer to help establish conformity. We see ourselves as in charge, and we believe we must never relinquish that responsibility. We expect the client to follow our lead and to be grateful we have assumed control and to do what we ask without question or delay. Our practice derives from these largely unquestioned beliefs once we decide clients differ from others and, consequently, are flawed.

By contrast, when we decide clients are people like us who need to sharply define goals to change and to draw upon and shape existing strengths to meet them, we create a different structure based on collaboration.[2] And, so, we experience our work quite differently. Just imagine how you would feel at the end of each workday if you viewed clients as collaborators needing help using their strengths to develop new skills. Enthusiastic, excited, and mentally stimulated describe the feelings that surface for me. Now, imagine how you would feel if you considered each and every client on your caseload flawed. Exhausted, frustrated, and anxious comes to mind. And our clients respond differentially as well. Those we consider collaborators become enthusiastic and participatory, while those we consider recipients become quietly or openly rebellious and frequently, lethargic.

It is possible to encounter adult clients, or even older children and teens requesting or being referred for therapy, who, because of their experience with previous therapists, educators, and other authority figures, such as parents, may resist the notion that, in relationship with an adult, they have anything to offer the enterprise than their compliant presence as scheduled. That is what I experienced with adult males with stuttering problems. They seemed to silently dare me to change them and became quite uncomfortable and resistant to taking on the role of Partner. Maybe they sensed that as Recipient they could resort to blaming the therapist when they did not change substantially, which may have been their ultimate goal, especially if they were playing the psychological Rescue Game.[3] When clients initially defer assuming the role of Partner, or collaborator, the therapist who prefers to Partner rather than to Rescue clients needs to focus on developing and closely monitoring a collaborative relationship with them or to decline to offer ongoing professional service.

So being practical becomes our standard. We recognize and accept what is, i.e., that clients, except for the comatose, can show us and collaborate with us to make the changes in their life they need and desire. Resisting this reality brings suffering to us both as we invest as much or more energy to establish our worthiness and self-righteousness rather than marshalling energy for expressed change. And that thought brings us to the next chapter, "Right and Wrong II: Harmonizing."

6 RIGHT AND WRONG II: HARMONIZING

"Do not search for the truth. Only cease cherishing your own thoughts

and opinions."

- - - T'sen T'sang, Zen Teacher

"When faced with choosing between being right and being kind, always choose being kind."

- - - Wayne Dyer (2007) citing Lao Tsu (1989)

On his nationally syndicated television show, psychologist Dr. Phillip McGraw, a.k.a "Dr. Phil," frequently asks adult participants, who insist on being right in their troubled relationships, *"Would you rather be happy or would you rather be right?"* That cryptically posed suggestion delivered with the authority and compassion of an experienced, skilled clinician bores through these somnambulant bullies' defensive shields, if only for a moment. As they hear these words, their torsos often crumple. Their chins typically lower. Their eyes often widen in sudden awareness. Then they typically pause momentarily to perhaps consider the possibility they may be winning at their chosen interpersonal game (Berne, 1996), but loosing significant relationships and their footing in life.

Dr. Phil may have invited these guests to his show because they represent so many of us determined to prove ourselves right at all times and, sometimes, at all costs. By publicly counseling them, he offers insight to many of us with similar orientations and the reasonable expectation that we, too, can learn healthier ways to interact with each other.

I'M RIGHT; YOU'RE WRONG. LOSE-LOSE

"Winning isn't the only thing; it's everything."

- - - Henry "Red" Sanders, UCLA football coach

The desire to be the one who is right seems rampant throughout our society: Consider political practices at any level of government and in any political party geared toward winning the next election; business practices that sacrifice customer service and employee care in a short-sighted effort to plump-up the bottom line; school board practices that flatly deny parent and citizen concerns at odds with standards and regulations; and, most importantly, family relationships characterized by endless bickering and antagonism over who is right and who is wrong. We want to prove we are right to feel good about ourselves, but do we? Do we act as though we are comfortable with ourselves, i.e., confident, generous when we win? Do we use our victory to help ourselves and others live happier, more satisfying lives? Or do we seize the next opportunity to again prove we are right as we continue our battle for mastery over others to satisfy some still unrecognized and unmet need inside us?

Most of us battle on. We seldom care whether or how we hurt one another. We seldom care who we hurt. Our partners, children, and colleagues or strangers in parking lots, ticket booths, or customer service positions can all become our victims.

Our sense of self-righteousness grows as we savor the fruit of winning, i.e. doing what we want while keeping others from doing what they want. We continue playing "I Win: You Loose," perhaps, with greater frequency and intensity. We carefully select players who we expect will crumple from our assault. If they surprise us with their strength, and we sense we may loose, we retreat. If we can not win, we will not allow someone to have victory over us. If the apparent winner is a friend, family member, or associate, who we can not easily avoid, we shut down when we need to be with them. We refuse to answer questions they ask, initiate conversation, or cooperate in any way. We are present but unavailable. In this way, we prevent them from having further victories over us while we maintain power over them by enticing them to play, "You Want Me More Than I Want You," a sub-game we are certain we can win.

Effect on Professional Practice

This seemingly addictive relational style is as prevalent in our profession as in our personal lives and in society- at-large. After all, what is a profession or a society than an extension of individual beliefs and related behaviors? If we, in our personal lives, thrive on being right, we will do so professionally. We will demand clients do as we say. When they disagree with our recommendations, we will do our best to convince them they are wrong, and we are right (e.g., Silverman, 2003c). If we fail to convince them through argumentation, we may refer them to someone else or provide treatment in a way that diminishes them and elevates our sense of self-righteousness. We may, for example, provide tasks and sequences of tasks which we believe they will find difficult, perhaps, impossible to successfully complete. We believe their failure will demonstrate to them just how right we are. That becomes our primary goal. Helping clients become the best they can be becomes a distant consideration. We are not interested in partnering with clients because we do not want to relate as equals. We prefer donning an authoritative role to intimidate clients into assuming a subordinate one.

We will demand colleagues think as we do if they wish to commune freely with us. If they advance points-of-view contrary to our own, we will snipe at them, more so if they had been especially close. For example, consider the chilling rift between Sigmund Freud, founder of psychoanalysis, and Carl Jung, his dearest disciple, when Jung decided to advance his analytic theory in opposition to Freud's assessment of the role of sexuality in human life and as an expression of his increasing interest in the role of the Unconscious. Their acrimonious break precipitated the creation of "camps" in the personal psychology community, which continues to this day. We, too, have "camps." They surface in classrooms presentations and discussions, seminars, textbooks, professional journals, workshops, and academic departments where students quickly learn to consider individuals who think as they and their instructors as right and those who think differently as wrong. Separating what instructors consider the intellectual wheat from the chaff, a prime function of training at the doctoral level, can be rationalized as paving the way for "newbies" to the profession to eventually secure membership in the right camp. We disregard the unfortunate effect encouraging such overt and implicit bickering has on students, the profession, and, ultimately, the public because all that really matters to us is that, individually, we are acknowledged as right We can see the fall-out from this unfortunate approach to education in the area of stuttering. Many students exposed to the magnitude of discord in the voluminous collection of experiential data and in the opinions of etiology, treatment, and maintenance become overwhelmed. They become doubtful they can sort through all the data to effectively treat children and adults with stuttering problems and often seek ways to avoid working with them. Some opt out of conducting research after witnessing occasional, violent ideological disputes erupt at research meetings.

As a graduate student in a research seminar on stuttering, I witnessed strong, strapping students become physically ill moments before class meetings conducted like an *ersatz* boot camp where the professor brutally forced us to admit we knew nothing about stuttering. Experiencing that intimidation led several to do research in other clinical areas. The professor's desire to be right, or to Search for the Truth, as he defined the process, required taking casualties. This instructional style may be acceptable in some venues, for instance, the armed forces and business, e.g., Bill Gates reportedly engaged in ". . . brutally breaking down employees in meetings."(Grossman, 2007), but it fails to model the skills students need to learn an egalitarian approach to clinical work or thoughtful research

Factions also develop in clinical settings in all venues, i.e., schools, outpatient and inpatient services, home health care, long-term health care, and private practice, but they operate somewhat more subtly and, perhaps, insidiously, since, as members of multidisciplinary teams, we are expected to, at least publicly, relate cooperatively with colleagues. Disagreements concerning clinical practice frequently become personalized and handled the way high-schoolers, who are clique members might. For instance, to borrow an example from business lore:

> *Two employees finishing lunch in the company cafeteria were reminiscing about employees no longer working for the company. Unexpectedly, one appears. The two call to their former colleague to invite him to sit with them. After a few preliminary remarks, he asks why they did not tell him they were unhappy working with him. Surprised at his candidness and by his awareness of their feelings about him as a co-worker, one mumbles, "We did not want to hurt your feelings." The other nods somberly in assent.*

Hearing that, the visitor leaps from his chair in animated disbelief at their apparent naïveté. He shouts, "Hurt My Feelings!? You got me fired! If you had told me I was using the wrong filing system, I could have changed that." He turns and stomps away.

The remaining two look briefly at each other, shrug their shoulders, and sigh, then resume their pre-visitation conversation.

Similarly, we therapists avoid confronting co-workers to whom we feel superior. Unlike academics, who frequently openly challenge colleagues and students whose ideas they believe inferior to their own, we tend to avoid direct confrontation. We occasionally are driven more by the need to be popular than the desire to seek the truth. We want to be regarded as nice, not as difficult. So, unwilling to relinquish our judgment that we are right and our colleagues wrong, we quietly avoid and exclude them to the extent allowed and withhold our support for their activities and projects. We see no personal value from sincere contact with colleagues who think differently than we.

Like politicians practicing doomed isolationist policies, we convince ourselves those who differ from us have nothing of value to share. But we know the real reason we wish to avoid those we consider inferior in their thinking and behavior is that they offend our sensibilities by suggesting we may be fallible, that we may be wrong. Our difference from them may make us wrong. Who knows? We keep our distance just in case. Perhaps, an added element of the historical change that President Barack Obama brings to the citizens of this country and the world is the value of associating closely and well with those holding divergent opinions. He believes doing so strengthens a leader.

POINT OF VIEW

Most undergraduates I taught preferred taking objective tests to essay examinations. They believed objective tests provide fairer assessments of their class knowledge than did essay examinations that evaluated their beliefs as well as their knowledge. They believed that, whereas, objective questions have only one correct answer even when a multiple-choice response may include two or more options, for instance insidious choice "D," which states: "A and B but not C," essay questions may generate several appropriate responses and degrees of development allowing the instructor the latitude to grade one acceptable answer higher than another. Objective questions, they argued, eliminated personal judgment by the scorer. What was right was right. No personal bias could creep in to lower their score, which is what they hoped to prevent. Of course, their argument was sound to a point: Parameters constituting a correct answer to an objective examination question are frequently more narrowly identified and readily verifiable than those applied to essay questions. But, given that their argument presumed *objective* implied universal and judgment-free, I felt compelled to share with them an experience provided by the instructor of the general semantics class I took as a graduate student. That experiment helped shape my life.

I invited the 30 or so class members of the introductory speech science course concerned about examination scorer reliability and validity to use a ruler I provided to measure the length of a line I had drawn on a 3" x 5" note card. I began by inquiring whether or not anyone present had not used a ruler to measure a line. This question never failed to garner brief and carefully masked stares of disbelief that an instructor of college students would even consider that unfamiliarity with the use of such an elementary measurement tool for such a common-place task was possible. I could sense their newly awoken curiosity wondering what would soon follow. I had their attention! At that point, I handed the card and ruler to a student in the front row and gave the instructions to measure the line, write its length on a slip of paper, pass the card and ruler to the person sitting behind them when done, and signal me when the last student had had an opportunity to complete the task. Then I launched into the day's scintillating lecture.

When informed all had had the opportunity to measure the line, I interrupted the lecture and directed that the slips of paper with their answers written on them be passed forward to a designated classmate. That person read aloud the answer on each slip of paper, one-by-one as I recorded each measurement on the chalkboard in the front of the room. Then I tallied the frequency of each answer. Within seconds, when it was clear there was no single answer to the seemingly simple, objective question, "How long is the line?" a stunned silence briefly settled over the class. After all, what could be simpler, what could be more objective than 30 people measuring the length of the same line with the same tool? Yet, even with that simple problem and the seemingly equivalent skill levels available to apply to the task, unanimity of measured length was not attained. In fact, in a class of 30 or so, three or four different measurements often surfaced.

When we considered the variables that may have contributed to the variance of the answer, such as body posture, visual acuity, and variations in lighting dependent seat location, most had developed a greater appreciation that an objective measure was a measure not without judgment. They learned what I hoped they would. Since then, of course, quantum mechanics has posited that no objectivity exists between an observer and the observed, further emphasizing the irrelevance of the concept "objective measurement."

Years later, when I was no longer involved in classroom teaching, I learned of the Buddhist Eightfold Path to Enlightenment. The very first step, Right View, immediately arrested my interest. As I considered what that might mean, I spontaneously imagined myself standing on an alpine-like mountainside viewing the valley below. Unlike Sister Maria of *The Sound of Music* fame, I was not twirling around in joyous wonderment celebrating the hills. I was standing very still and looking with interest at the picturesque valley below. Others around me quietly seemed to be observing the same scene. Without forethought, my ever-present sense of competition and my experience with photography simultaneously informed the experience, and I instantly realized no two of us could see the valley in quite the same way. We would not literally see it the same way, and we would not comprehend it the same way. That stark realization gave fresh meaning to my use of the phrase Point-of-View from then on. Previously, I used the phrase dismissively to convey the lack of gravity I considered one person's opinion to contain, as in, *"Well, that is just your point-of-view."* with my tone of voice and phrasing emphasizing the word *just*, signifying that while they were entitled to express their opinion the way an unskilled and unprepared horse may be allowed to run a race by virtue of paying an entrance fee, no one would want to bet on it. Personal opinions had validity but limited usefulness. Now, I see and value them in both my personal and professional exchanges as windows into the experience of others.

Because we can not occupy the same location with another, we can not expect to share an identical view. That was the lesson I learned from contemplating the meaning of Right View. But even if we could, our own two eyes might not register the same view when focused on an object. For instance, when we hold up object, say, a pen, at arms' length and focus on it with both eyes, we see it in a particular location. But, if we then close one eye and look at it again, we may see it in a different place, even though we did not perceptibly move our arm or hand between views. If our left eye is dominant, we see the pen an inch or so off to the left when we look at it with our right eye. It appears where it was when we look once again with only our left eye. If our right eye is dominant, and we look at it only with that eye, we will see the pen where we saw it when we looked at it with both eyes. But, when we look at it only with our left eye, it appears to have shifted to the right. This binocular reality suggests an alternative meaning to the old saw, *"The right hand does not know what the left hand is doing."* The two eyes see differently, irrespective of their individual acuity. So, which eye's image is right and which eye's image is wrong? Of course, neither one's is right nor is neither one's wrong. Each is dependent on variables which affect our two eyes differently and the concepts of "right" and "wrong" do no apply. As a matter of fact, one could argue they never do. All is a matter of Point-of-View. To insist, that one position is "right" and another is "wrong" is to encourage the type of argumentation that creates angry and acrimonious feelings and behavior. That can fuel the sort of mindset that leads to the waging of war, nationally and professionally.

What Does Anger Have To Do With It?

According to an ancient Buddhist fable, certain of the Buddha's disciples were disturbed by the discord traveling scholars and seers were creating among the people by popularizing polarizing views about life. Some were insisting the world was finite and eternal while others were declaring it was neither finite nor eternal. Some claimed the soul died with the body while others said the soul lived on forever. Their opinions generated all matter of disagreement. Concerned about the disharmony they generated, the disciples decided to ask the Buddha what was true. In response, the Buddha told the following story about a *raja,* several blind men, and an elephant:

> *A raja invited the blind men of the town to his palace. When the men assembled, he instructed his servant to introduce them individually to an elephant. The servant positioned one alongside the elephant's head and said, "This is an elephant." He positioned one next to the elephant's tail and said, "This is an elephant." He placed one next to the trunk and said, "This is an elephant." and so on, until all the men had an opportunity to see the elephant in this way. When they reassembled, the raja asked them, "What sort of thing is the elephant?" The one who saw the head replied the elephant was like a pot. The one who saw the tail said the elephant was like a pestle. The one who saw the trunk insisted the elephant was like a plough. And so on.*
>
> *A great argument ensued among the blind me, punctuated by blows. Each man insisted what he knew to be the only truth.*

The Buddha explained to his disciples that the scholars and seers were like the blind men. They confused the segment of reality they knew with the whole. Clinging to their views, they created dogmas. And, because they were of a quarrelsome nature, they fought to maintain their beliefs.

The truth is we are like the blind men of the fable. We have a tendency to fight for the supremacy of our views over the views of others based on our knowledge, which, like the blind men's, is only part of the whole. And, like the blind men, we too fail to know and appreciate that which we know and believe to be true is only a part of that which is true. Look around the earth. Consider the situation in the Middle East, in various regions of Africa, in the Balkans, and elsewhere. Consider the political in-fighting in this country and others. And Consider the behavior of professionals, in speech and hearing and other areas, when unexpected ideas are presented or unpopular views championed in the classroom, in journals, at conferences, and at work. Take a moment to visualize the faces of those who react with disapproval. See the anger, the hostility, the apparent disregard for the welfare of those "on the other side." Study those faces! Under similar circumstances, they can be our own. Most of us have such a hard time expanding our world view beyond our own hold on reality that we would rather fight to the death, if need be, than open our minds. American Buddhist nun, Pema Chödrön's (2005c) humorous account of an angry situation highlights the irony of this sorry aspect of our functioning:

> A peace demonstration was underway in a large city when some of onlookers began physically assaulting the marchers. The marchers, in response, hit the onlookers over their heads with their peace signs.

When we think we hold the right opinion on a matter and another holds the wrong one, we can get so angry at the other we become momentarily insane. Engulfed by anger, we lack reason, and we can become capable of causing great harm to ourselves and others. That is when we need to stop what we are thinking and stop what we are doing and center ourselves. Once we settle down by breathing with awareness for 10 or 12 consecutive breaths or engaging in another form of mindful activity for 10 or more consecutive minutes, such as walking meditation (e.g., Hanh, 2004), we can contemplate why it is that another's point-of-view, different from our own, can make us so angry. When we do, we may realize reality may be greater than we had realized. Acknowledging that begs the conclusion we will need to enlarge our view of ourselves, others, and the world around us to live with integrity. That awareness can be very frightening. It can shake the ground on which we stand because it erases some of the predictability of our daily lives. Even though we may complain are lives are a bit repetitive and boring, we crave the security that apparent predictability brings. If we embrace our new, greater view of life, we realize we will lose at least some of our certainties, and we will need to change how we live (e.g., Silverman, 2007). That is why pioneers in all realms face antagonism and censure, even death. Their discoveries beg for elemental change. For those of us terrified by the need to make basic life changes, we may react with great anger because being angry seems more comfortable than facing and dealing with our fear.[1]

As we continue to examine the reason for our anger at another for holding a belief different from our own, we may make yet another startling discovery: We and the person who seems to think so differently from us really thinks as we do. We became angry with her because we thought she was close-minded and hard-hearted, and she became angry with us because she thought *we* were close-minded and hard-hearted. Then we discover: There is no basis for taking sides! There is no basis for fighting. We are basically the same. We each want to have our own way and expect the other to willingly embrace it. As we look deeper, we discover in essence, we want something even more elemental, i.e., what is best for ourselves and for others. So, recognizing that our similarity is stronger than our difference, we can begin to problem-solve to get what we each want (e.g., Rosenberg, 2003).

Causes and Solutions

When we come to look more deeply at ourselves and our problems, we begin to realize that fundamentally the conditions that challenge us have similar causes, i.e., provocations and our response to it, but different personal solutions. For instance, many of us find accepting our body image difficult. We think we are too fat, so we diet and exercise, meditate and visualize to become toned and fit so we can look good and wear the clothes we wish, or not wear clothes if we wish. Like me, many have tried several different methods to look trim and fit. We may have tried a series of fad diets, like the low-carbohydrate diet, the all protein diet, the grapefruit diet, the liquid diet, the lettuce diet, and so on. We may have entered a professional program to loose weight by eating their specially prepared food and following their daily regime. We may have counted calories or adopted a reduced calorie diet, measured portion size, attended to food category, become vegetarian, restricted our intake to raw food, and so forth. We may even have opted for a surgical procedure to help us jump-start our loss of excess body weight. We eventually learned we needed to incorporate a program of daily activity with our diet change to encourage our bodies to release the extra bulk they carried. Cardio work, stretching, weight-lifting, walking more, and combinations of these helped move us toward our goal. Then, we became wiser. We acknowledged to ourselves that to look as we wish we would need to stop sporadic dieting and make a life-long commitment to healthier living. We needed to eat the healthiest food in appropriate amounts, stop emotional eating by learning to recognize and meet our emotional needs in direct and healthy ways, and work our bodies daily. So, while the causes of being overweight are similar from person to person, i.e., moving little and eating unhealthy food to excess, the solution for each of us individually can vary considerably as we make personal choices regarding diet, exercise, surgical intervention, and meeting our emotional needs. And the timing and combination of the methods we choose further personalize our individual approaches. No one's plan is everyone's choice or need. No one's goal is everyone's. There is no need to fight over which method is right for everyone. We only need to select the plan that is right for us personally.

We similarly address other personal needs, such as dealing with chronic pain, various forms of cancer, baldness, stuttering, accent reduction, dysphagia, and so on. We select methods and programs consistent with our temperament, spirituality, lifestyle, health, and culture then balance them with accessibility, cost, and family needs to develop an individual plan. This way we can create many so-called right programs. As an example, consider treatment for stuttering problems. Problems of stuttering share essentially two co-dependent causes: The first is the trigger for stuttering itself, when stuttering was an unanticipated interrupter of the flow of speech, such as repetition, insertion of sound and syllable, silent pause, and the like. And the second is our response to that experience of stuttering, i.e., how we interpreted what it meant for us to stutter and what we think we should do about it (e.g., Bloodstein, 1995). From personal experience, I can remember thinking as a young child that because I stuttered I could not talk right. I was three at the time I first became aware I was stuttering, and I attended to two aspects of the experience: 1) How it felt to me and 2) How my mother responded when I stuttered. I panicked as I stuttered because I felt I was losing control of my body. That was when my mother became my interpreter to shield me from the need to talk. She provided what I needed when I wanted it and provided it *before I asked*. I recall feeling profound relief that she made it possible for me to not talk. I also felt awestruck that she was able to know what I thought. After she died suddenly when I was three and one-half and no one stepped in to fill the void she left in my life, I eventually chose to be selectively mute (Silverman, 2003d).

How we help someone with a distinct or emerging stuttering problem involves choosing among multiple intervention possibilities. Even though the original provocation for stuttering may be quite similar for each of us, i.e., genetic inheritance, language learning, communication skill learning (e.g., Silverman, 1970), the way stuttering problems surface and evolve depends more on the influence of individual circumstances, such as temperament, family structure, cultural and societal values, and experience with speech therapy (e.g., Silverman, 2001a). Issues such as these that foster and maintain stuttering problems need to be addressed individually in a meaningful combination and sequence. So, it seems that to improve our clinical effectiveness with individuals with stuttering problems and those who care for them, we can better spend our time, talent, and energy sharing the interventions we know from personal experience to have helped those with whom we have worked as well as those approaches which do not seem to have been helpful, rather than arguing about which is the right solution.

Arguing about which is the right treatment is no more worthwhile use of our time and energy and no more beneficial to those with stuttering problems than it is for physicians, dieticians, personal trainers, and life coaches to argue about which weight loss approach is right for all. As I write these lines, I recall one of the final scenes from the movie, "The Last Samurai" (2003). During his life, the leader of the few remaining *samurai* in Japan searched for the perfect cherry blossom. That was to become his enduring spiritual quest that seemed unfulfilled. But, as he lay dying from wounds he received fighting for the honor of the *samurai* tradition against the Japanese Emperor's forces determined to eradicate this pivotal social class, the warrior reflected on the many blossoms he had seen. Then, with surprise, awe, and relief, he vocalized his sudden awareness, *"They are all perfect."* and died peacefully. His deathbed declaration that all cherry blossoms are perfect seemed to be his doorway from life to death, one he seemed to gratefully enter. If we can reach the awareness that one helpful intervention to prevent someone from developing or overcoming a problem is no better or no worse than another, then, like the *samurai*, we too will be able to find our peace.

COMING TOGETHER

Sometimes, during an argument, when participants cling to their points-of-view as right and view divergent one's as wrong, an onlooker or one of the argumentative parties themselves suggests: *"Let's agree to disagree."* Appreciating the inherent sanity expressed in those five words that encourages those involved to seek harmony rather than perpetuate the current disharmony, individuals often stop, disengage from their self-manufactured gridlock and begin more effective discussion or separate for a time. They seem willing to consider it is not possible or, even, necessary for each of them to hold the same opinion to resolve what seems to be causing them to be at odds with one another.

We, too, can experience such seemingly dead-end conflicts at staffings, conferences, and day-to-day exchanges when we express our point-of-view about a matter, and someone else, a colleague, client, or caregiver, presents a seemingly different one. And that is when we can benefit all involved by suggesting that we *agree to disagree.* This will do more toward bringing us together in common cause than mindlessly following the unfortunate impulse so many of us have at these times of trying to persuade clients and caregivers we are right and they are wrong. Arguing others down is what we are likely to do when we are relatively inexperienced and fresh from school. As a student, we customarily learn to fear being wrong as a practical consideration. We want to graduate and help others by making what teachers, clinical staff, and, even, other students consider the right decisions and execute treatment plans in the right way. Once we have graduated and successfully completed our clinical fellowship year, we still may be strongly motivated in our decisions and actions by the fear of being wrong. We have heard about the possibility of facing malpractice litigation, and we believe colleagues and clients will always judge us. We realize we need to be right in our decisions and actions to establish a respected and long-lived career. So, when we experience the inevitable differences of opinion with clients and caregivers that arise, we may believe we need to convince them we are in the right. We may even believe that we are responsible to educate clients, caregivers, and, even, colleagues to think as we do. If we believe all that and if we are inexperienced and lacking in knowledge about how best to relate professionally, we may take the path of argumentation to resolve seeming differences (e.g., Charon, 2006; Silverman, 2003c).

We may feel good about our chosen interaction style if we observe that a vigorous and sometimes stern presentation of our beliefs and recommendations squelches opposition on-the-spot so that we can move forward without untoward delay. But, often, there comes a time when, during the course of our working together, clients and caregivers simply give up on achieving what they want with our help. They show up, but they do so by metaphorically dragging their heels. They come late. They come without evidence of having practiced their newly developing skills. They are present in body, not in spirit, until they quit or we dismiss them for lack of progress.

After observing this disturbing pattern repeat, we feel increasingly depressed and angry. We take our work seriously. We long to feel satisfaction from helping others doing what we do. But being rejected leaves us feeling unappreciated, unsuccessful, and angry especially since we know we showed in every way we knew that we cared. And we believe we offered our skills unstintingly. Feeling unsuccessful, we despair continuing to work if this is our payoff for all our concern and care. Yet we believe this is the work we want to do. We realize something needs to change. Initially, we may decide to learn new skills to work with a treatment population other than the one which seems not to appreciate our work. For instance, we may learn to perform bedside and modified barium swallow evaluations and treatment skills to help people with swallowing difficulties swallow more safely and effectively rather than continue to work with individuals recovering from traumatic brain injury, who we have found to be too questioning and too argumentative. Making that change to take on a new challenge may lead us to feel enthusiastic about our day-to-day work once again. The welcome perkiness in our manner and freshness in our outlook we relish may continue for some time. Then, when our new responsibilities become routine, we may once again experience colleagues appearing to shirk from or limit exchanges with us and clients behaving unenthusiastically as they work with us. Taking the time to calmly reflect upon this unexpected and disappointing circumstance, we may come to understand that to experience a satisfying work environment we will need to do more than to develop new technical skills. After all, we are the common link between the discomforting experience we had working with adults with traumatic brain injury and the unpleasant one emerging as we work with adults experiencing *dyspagia*. The technical skills we apply differ from one situation to the next, but we notice we are going about our new job the same way we did our old one. We courageously acknowledge to ourselves that our tendency to want to be right and our willingness to argue those who disagree with us into apparent submission is causing our unhappiness. That is what is driving clients, caregivers, and colleagues into silent resistance and is draining the atmosphere of creative potential. That is what is causing our dissatisfaction with work. Quietly, yet joyfully, we realize, as did the title character of the comic strip, Pogo, when he studied his image in a full-length mirror that, *"We have met the enemy and he is us"* (Kelly, 1987). Now we know what will help.

Ironically, we know from our study of human history and individual and group psychology that human nature relishes autonomy. We do. Yet, we frequently interact with clients and caregivers as though, in this particular relationship, that consideration does not apply to them. We tell ourselves we all will profit from a win-win experience if we adopt a dominant role and assign clients and caregivers a submissive one. And, then, that is how we arrange our clinical relationships. As though we were children inviting another child to play during recess at school, we metaphorically shout: *"I'll be leader, and you'll be follower."* For example, we introduce ourselves to the adult clients we address as "Sam" or "Max" or "My Man," as "Susan Lightower," "Ms. Lightower," or "Dr. Lightower." We wear white lab coats. We sit at our desk in an upholstered chair and invite them to occupy an armless, plastic one. We take personal and business calls and tolerate interruptions from professional and support staff but expect them to turn off their cell phones during their scheduled time with us. At the end of our appointment, we offer them our business cards.

If clients are of preschool or school age, we expect them to follow our rules and enthusiastically engage in our customs because we envision our interactions with them as occurring within our world, which they have entered as our invited or tolerated guests. If they fail to abide by our laws and traditions, we often send them away rather than negotiate more personally meaningful and mutually acceptable rules of engagement (e.g., Rosenberg, 2004). Or, if we prefer their world to our own or believe that by appearing as if we do we are more likely to lure them into achieving goals we set for them, we may adopt some of their behaviors. We do so to create the impression, despite our chronological age difference, we relate similarly to the world and are interested in being friends. We may, for instance, dress similarly by wearing the latest fad items, such as gel shoes, jeans, Dr. Who tee-shirts, friendship bracelets, flower rings, etc. We may adopt their *lingo*, their walk, and their interests. We hope, by aping them, they will think we and they are one and feel they can trust us without risk. But by blurring adult-child boundaries, we risk creating the ultimate relationship turn-off with youthful clients typically disdainful of older people struggling to win their acceptance. We also risk causing emotional chaos (e.g., Chess and Thomas, 2005) for them and us by suggesting we are what we are not. In successful relationships, all parties experience autonomy on their own terms (e.g., Rosenberg, 2003).

Children and adults, who have come to expect a care provider or an educator to dominate them, usually quietly acquiesce when we verbally and nonverbally announce that the rules of engagement with us require playing "The Big Boss" and that we will be "The Big Boss." When they receive this message, some immediately rebel, some become passive and remain passive, and some seem cooperative until they, too, rebel, subtly at first, and, eventually, strongly if we seem to ignore their early expressions of dissatisfaction interacting with us. Client and caregiver rebellion usually surprises us, and we may feel angry, hurt, and scared, in any combination, facing rejection. At first, we may be shocked. We failed to notice, pre-occupied as we were achieving our goals for them, that although they may have deigned to play, they did so resentfully because they believed they had no choice. We forgot that even infants appreciate the opportunity for direct, personal expression, as studies of baby signing demonstrate (e.g., Acredolo and Goodwyn, 1996). When hearing babies learn manual signing, they no longer depend on caregivers' guesswork to decipher the meaning of their sounds, posture, and movements. Infants and toddlers who sign to caregivers until they learn to speak become happier and more content than those who do not. And their caregivers reportedly experience more satisfaction and happiness interacting with them than do caregivers of infants and toddlers who do not communicate through sign.

As our sense of shock subsides and our feelings of anger, resentment, and, possibly, bitterness diminish, we acknowledge their rebellion was a fierce demand to be heard. We like to think that by asking questions, administering tests, designing tasks to develop and hone skills, and offering information and advice we did all we could as professionals. But, when we consider our own experiences seeking help, we know we personally want more than being advised, observed, probed, prodded, and questioned (e.g., Charon, 2006; Silverman, 2004; Silverman, 2003a). We want to partner with someone we feel knows us, someone who understands our needs and has the capacity to help us meet them, someone who engages us in telling our stories of challenges and opportunities for release. So do our clients and caregivers.

Filial Imprinting

I believe we tend to dismiss what we personally know about the importance of fully engaging clients and caregivers in the process of facing their life challenges with the curiosity, confidence, and enthusiasm partnering encourages because of the *filial imprinting* (e.g., Kisilevsky *et. al*, 2003; Lorenz and Kickert, 2004) we experience as students and young professionals. Filial imprinting occurs when, as neophytes, we intuitively claim seasoned professionals in our immediate environment as role models and adopt their behavior as our standard of professional conduct. This passive learning, which occurs during the most sensitive and vulnerable phase of our development as professionals, can be difficult to reverse (e.g., Lorenz and Kickert, 2004).

We become imprinted by faculty, clinical staff, off-site supervisors, and, even, more advanced students. Having no other practical and meaningful way to learn how to be a speech-language pathologist, we watch them work with clients and caregivers and interact with each other. We study their decision-making processes. We consider their relational styles, noting carefully their use of language, speech, and voice, how and when they touch clients and caregivers, and their spatial positioning, or *proxemics*, as they work. And we analyze their manner of dress and grooming. Some of their behaviors and their reasoning processes appear so appealing we almost immediately decide to incorporate them. Others may not draw our admiration or coincide with our evolving clinical point-of-view, but faculty and clinical staff expect us to adopt them, at least on the premises, to experience using them. In the former circumstance, when we adopt what we consider admirable behaviors and beliefs, we believe we are behaving at the highest level of which we believe we are capable. In the latter, when we adopt required behaviors and beliefs, we are doing what is simply expected. In either circumstance, we usually believe, by emulating these beliefs and practices, our own clinical practice is made sound.

We may know we may be a little rough around the edges as we incorporate these specific skills into our professional *persona*. We may know we may not look as sharp using them as those we are emulating. But we are not terribly concerned. We believe, with time and with practice, we will function smoothly, like those who have gone before us. And we believe we are learning how to do things right. Those beliefs are what gives us confidence to enter the profession as fledglings and, in a circular way, often causes us to cling almost desperately to them. We consider them our lifeline to sure footing. We hold to them as the ground, or matrix of our professional *persona*. While we continue to develop skills and competencies for eliciting, rewarding, and nourishing behaviors and for responding effectively to our feelings and those of our clients and their caregivers, students and colleagues as we go along, we generally hold quite fiercely to our core beliefs of what it means to be a speech-language pathologist and how to relate as one. After all, those very beliefs helped us graduate from school, complete our clinical fellowship year, and find work as professionals. Few of us will relinquish what we consider the core of our identity and success. As long as they seem to be working for us, we have no inclination to let them go. So, if we were imprinted with the belief that effective clinicians assume an authoritative role with clients, caregivers, students, and colleagues, we will more than likely assume that role ourselves. Since many of our colleagues have been imprinted as have we, it may take quite some time for us to recognize the value to us and to those with whom we work of switching to an egalitarian model of clinical service. And it may take considerable courage to enact the change once we recognize the value of making it since doing so probably will mean we will need to go against the current, proverbial tide. As a personal example, I experienced considerable opposition when, in 1980, I petitioned to develop and teach a course in counseling skills for graduate and undergraduate speech-language pathology majors in the department where I had taught for several years.

> *When I undertook Transactional Analysis (TA) training to complement the clinical skills I was using, I came to believe the partnering model championed in TA was more effective for more clients than the authoritarian one I had been taught to use. I also realized the clinical skills I was learning as a TA trainee could help other speech-language pathologists develop into more effective clinicians. So I petitioned the departmental faculty where I was teaching to allow me to develop and teach a course in counseling theory and methodology. The department chair was hesitant to approve my request because there was insufficient support for the idea among the faculty, all of whom considered themselves clinicians. As one faculty member said to me, "We don't need a course in counseling. Our students aren't going to be counselors!" Nevertheless, the department chair forwarded my request to the College Dean, who also happened to be a speech-language pathologist in an earlier incarnation. He apparently planned to refuse my request for the same reasons as the majority of faculty, but, before he announced his decision, he consulted with the director of the campus counseling program. He expected the director to view a course in counseling offered by different campus unit an invasion of his professional territory so that he would object to offering the course I was proposing. But, to his surprise, the director*

encouraged the course as a desirable curriculum addition. He apparently said, "We need all the courses in counseling we can offer."

So, I was allowed to develop and teach a course on counseling for speech-language pathology majors, but, throughout the four years I taught it, faculty in the department remained coolly disdainful and rarely recommended it to students. During the many years I had taught in the department, many of the faculty demonstrated a low tolerance for personal and professional change, which, like most of us, they seemed to find threatening. The course in counseling frightened those faculty and staff who recognized it could shatter their accustomed concept of the profession and their approach to teaching it, so they resisted the course with all their might. Such a response is not unusual to a new idea, but since I thought it was such a right idea, so obvious a plus to the curriculum, I, relatively young and inexperienced initiating radical change, became surprised, impatient, then deeply angered by the forms and strength of resistance I received by the majority of the faculty. I melted into a pool of self-righteous hurt. Despite having earned academic tenure, I quit to escape the pain I felt as an out-numbered member of a very testy coalescence to locate peace and happiness somewhere else.

"I'm Right; You're Wrong." was what we were playing. What a waste of time! What a waste of energy! And what a poor example of conflict resolution to offer students! I did not know that then. But I do now. I genuinely regret my colleagues and I were unable to find a way to amicably agree to disagree. And I am quite aware that my beliefs about right and wrong contributed mightily to the sorry circumstance. I since have learned the relativity of right and wrong and that peace and happiness come from within. If you do not find it there, you will not find it anywhere. As the founder of the increasingly popular mindfulness based stress reduction program (MBSR) Dr. Jon Kabat-Zinn (1995) entitled one of his books, *Wherever You Go There You Are.*

A "By the Way"

The department I left was not unique in its unwillingness to incorporate counseling course into its speech-language pathology curriculum. That belief was fairly commonplace in the late '70's, but it is one that is weakening slightly, as the increasing number of textbooks on counseling suggests. Clinicians value tools and skills for developing effective relationships with clients, caregivers, students, and colleagues. Many realize the relationship they cultivate with clients and caregivers is their most important tool (Silverman, 2006b) and they need direction to help create functional ones because relying exclusively on life experience is not sufficient. For instance, even in 1992, when I taught an early morning mini-seminar on incorporating counseling skills into clinical practice at the ASHA Convention (Silverman, 1992) more than 1,000 attendees jammed the room where the course was scheduled to be taught, a room able to seat a maximum of 500 to 600 people. I would not be surprised to see those who structure curricula increasingly incorporate instruction in counseling into the academic mix. That is my point-of-view.

PART III

ESTABLISHING CHANGE

When we embrace a sound plan for change, we need to apply substantial amounts of patience and endurance to the work. By committing to the plan for as long as it takes, we can more readily overcome the temptation to think and act as we have and less likely to succumb to the false belief that change lies beyond our grasp as we encounter inevitable obstacles. To succeed in a process fraught with emotional whirlpools and eddies of varying size, duration, and depth requires us to conserve, amplify, and regenerate our energy. That necessitates slowing down our level of physical and mental activity to function mindfully. Slowing down helps us develop space and flexibility to grow insights and skills needed for change.

7 SLOWING DOWN TO STRENGTHEN ENDURANCE[1]

PATIENCE AND SKILL-BUILDING

There is a certain performance skill common to golf, tennis, and other sports, and it is named *Follow-Through*. When we hit a golf ball off a tee, from a fairway, or out of a rough or bunker, pro's tell us to complete our swing to help send it where we want it to go before we observe the ball's path. Likewise, when we serve or volley playing tennis, we will be more likely to hit a winner if we finish the stroke before tracking its trajectory. Impatience to know where the ball is headed before completing the stroke adversely affects where it lands. Similarly, when a football wide receiver or special teams player runs for the end zone before catching and securing the football, fumbling becomes a real threat. Taking it where he wants it to go is only possible after catching the ball.

I first seriously considered the importance of finishing well when I studied classical guitar as a middle-aged adult. Among the many challenges I personally faced was learning to follow through on each finger stroke. My incredibly patient teacher emphasized that a good ending is as important as a good beginning and that was what I needed to learn. He explained I ended each stroke as I touched the string rather than following through by extending my finger a slight distance beyond it. By failing to follow through, I sacrificed a full, rich sound for a duller one. As I absorbed his instruction, I realized the way I stroked guitar strings was the way I lived. I gave fairly detailed thought about starting personal and business relationships but not how to end them. When I felt the need to end a relationship, I left. I attended to legal considerations, if any, and then moved on, as I had been taught as a child. I repressed the hurt, anger, and, often, the quality of the relationship itself that encouraged me to cut and run from unpleasantness. My guitar teacher helped me see that endings are part of a momentum, not an after-thought. While I never learned to play well enough to keep my cat from running screaming from the room when I practiced, I did feel satisfied I was learning how to create a more pleasing sound and a better life!

Another important lesson I learned from my guitar teacher's teaching was that the quality of endings influences the quality of beginnings. If, in writing, for example, we share what we know as thoroughly and as well as we know how for the intended reader to benefit from our experience and analysis, we will feel satisfied when we have written the last word on the last page. Then we probably will approach our next writing project with heightened confidence and more eagerness than trepidation. Likewise, when we conclude clinical programs, research projects, or formal teaching assignments planned with genuine consideration for how to structure them to best affect the lives of clients, students, and colleagues, we can feel a sense of satisfaction that generates excitement within us when we again approach these same sorts of tasks.

With the role of endings as portals to beginnings in mind, I have chosen to address endurance, which I associate with patience, as the subject of this, the final chapter of *Mind Matters,* because bringing to fruition suggestions made in earlier chapters requires endurance and considerable patience. Centuries ago, Saint Frances de Sales, a Roman Catholic cleric, reportedly advised those seeking personal change by saying: *"What is needed is a cup of understanding, a barrel of love, and an ocean of patience."* Contemporaneously, publication of a collection of Mother Teresa's letters to her spiritual confessors and her superior stunningly reveal that she, who many already consider a saint, suffered quietly yet tremendously for decades from what she perceived as a lack of communion with Jesus (Mother Teresa and Brian Kolodiejchuk, 2007). Having experienced an apparently authentic mystical communion with Jesus as a young nun that led her to minister to the *"poorest of the poor"* in Calcutta, she came to feel despair from lack of a felt sense of Jesus' presence personally and in the *eucharist*, something members of her religious community claim never to have sensed. Yet she persevered. She continued what she believed to be her work for Him until failing health and, then, death itself stopped her. Her determination and persistence in the absence of recognizable personal reward personifies not only faith but endurance. Mother Teresa made a commitment and patiently kept it. In the process, she created a structure that magnified her original efforts and continues to grow. But, perhaps, new knowledge of her enduring patience may have a transformative effect on countless more lives than the actual missionary work itself.

Many of us find patience a challenge when committing to change. Once we decide we want to look and act differently, we want to see the results we anticipate quickly, sometimes the next day. For instance, during my undergraduate clinical training in stuttering problems, I encountered a woman with a stuttering problem who had achieved a certain notoriety at our university speech clinic. Monica, a woman in her mid-30's, single, and employed as a secretary in a large organization, enrolled in therapy to address her severe stuttering problem. Within a short time, she accurately demonstrated Van Riper's (1973) control techniques. But, to the student clinicians' and supervisors' befuddlement, mild annoyance, and controlled amusement, she would use them only behind treatment doors because, she explained, *"They don't feel natural."* Somehow, Monica had not been advised or had rejected the suggestion that she practice them daily for an extended period in various and graded situations for them to feel natural. The controls were new behaviors. Until she habituated to them as she might a new pair of hiking boots, she would feel slightly awkward and, even, uncomfortable, as she might with new boots. Until Monica took time to successfully integrate these speech tools into her daily life through patient practice, they could not feel "natural."

In my late 20's and early 30's, I, too, wanted immediate results without doing the required work. I wanted to lose weight, and I wanted to do it quickly without feeling hunger. So I would quit the day after I began a diet or the day after that if I had not lost a pound or two! I would justify this short-lived diet by telling myself I was a big-boned woman fated to be heavy and that hunger from dieting was an unnecessary burden for me. Then, I would console myself with greasy foods and sweets to salve my hurt feelings at having deprived myself of food I loved and for my genuine disappointment at not having lost weight. After a while, the misery of being fat once again exceeded the anticipated agony of dieting, so, like someone fearful of diving into a river, I screwed up my courage then jumped into another diet. I repeated this sorry cycle several times during those years. Later, I finally overcame my diet-related impatience by learning what was required to successfully lose weight. I counted calories and exercised regularly. And I reframed my self-talk and feelings about eating and dieting. When I felt hungry or deprived or my weight plateaued, I reminded myself how good I would look and feel if I continued to eat and exercise appropriately. I reminded myself that as I continued to consume fewer calories than I burned, my body would, of necessity, lose unnecessary weight, at a pace appropriate for it. And I reminded myself of the shame and disappointment I would experience if I did not continue with this dietary and lifestyle change to achieve my goals. I learned to apply patience to the process through such self-talk and steely commitment,

Changing requires patience with the process, something our "fast food," "breaking news," "instant credit," and "texting" culture and, perhaps, our hard-wiring makes difficult by strongly and insistently, overtly and subliminally urging us to seek instant gratification. For example, we want the tools we can learn to use to manage our stuttering to create natural-feeling, fluent speech in all circumstances shortly after first trying them, our hearing aids to integrate seamlessly with our lifestyle once we purchase them, and our voice to project clearly and effortlessly throughout three consecutive hours of lecturing days after surgery to remove nodules on our vocal folds, even when we know better.

Impatience frequently leads clients to quit therapy when they fail to achieve personal goals according to their own timetables, as I stopping dieting after one or two days of eating sensibly because I failed to loose weight. Unfortunately, when clients do that, they frequently exempt themselves from responsibility for failing to achieve their goals, as I did when I precipitously stopped dieting because blaming someone or something felt more comfortable than taking personal responsibility. They are apt to tell themselves:

A) Speech therapy does not work.

B) The speech therapist was unhelpful. And/or

C) They can not change.

Such conclusions spurred by impatience, fueled by lack of or inadequate information and, perhaps, as contradictory as it may seem, fear of actual change (e.g., Silverman, 2007a) generate far-reaching and harmful effects. They may discourage further work for personal change and, when expressed to others, may discourage or delay them from seeking therapy or recommending it. Moreover, they may shake the confidence of newly certified speech-language pathologists, who, in the early stage of their careers, may, at least tacitly, doubt whether or not therapy works. The up-side is that by deeply contemplating such disruptive reactions to the therapy they provide, beginning therapists may come to realize that our job is not to "fix" clients (e.g., SpillIers, 2007). Our job is to help clients and caregivers change, which we are in a stronger position to accomplish when we conceptualize our role as "Partner" rather than "Rescuer" (Please See Chapter 2, "Partnering, Yes. Rescuing, No.").

The Fruits of Patience

We can not underestimate the role patience plays in the change process for both clients and caregivers. Patience is second only in importance to accurate knowledge about what may be involved and what is required. Of course, patience does not constitute passive idleness. In successful treatment, as in Mother Teresa's uniquely effective and inspiring work, steadfast persistence and endurance supports our work and permits the fruits of our labors to ripen as they will. As we cultivate patience, we, as helpers:

- *Respond with understanding and kindness rather than reacting with knee-jerk irritation or hurt to what displeases us.*

- *Recall and maintain our sense of identity and purpose.*

- *Recognize our inter-connection with those with whom we work.*

Let us briefly consider each in turn:

1) *Choosing our response to what displeases us.* In which, if any, of the following *scenarios* would you find it difficult to make the required decisions calmly and thoughtfully:

> A. Learning, during your morning break, you need to prepare three student treatment plans by the end of an already full day

> B. Unexpectedly being requested by the school principal to confer with parents of a newly enrolled student before you leave school that day

> C. Receiving a request from your supervisor to submit a list of materials and supplies when you arrive the next morning

> D. Hearing from the clinic administrator that your request for funding to create a waiting room for children separate from the one used by adults was once again denied unless you submit convincing statistics at next month's board meeting scheduled for next week that clinic revenue will benefit from such physical alteration to the facility

These not so atypical situations cause many of us to gnash our teeth and pull our hair and, perhaps, want to disappear. We feel irritated and annoyed as a reaction to our fear we can not perform as our personal professional standards demand without time and financial resources to do so. And, yet, that is the reality of the work-a-day world for many of us. We feel we are asked to do too much with too little, and we feel forced to comply with job requirements by reluctantly compromising or sacrificing our values. We know responding with irritation and anger diminishes our effectiveness by piling stress on others and further stressing us. But we are angry and losing patience. *What are we to do?*

2) *Recalling why we have chosen to do this work.* Paperwork demands increase exponentially yearly, or so it seems. Evaluation reports. Progress reports. Staffing reports. Daily notes. All this writing can snuff out our passion. Few, if any, of us became therapists to spend so much of our work days writing for third parties. Yet, we know that these forms of written communication can tightly focus our interventions and amplify the effectiveness of our patient contact time, but we realize the time required to successfully complete paper work requires us to spend increasingly more personal time keeping up with information and trends reported in professional journals, textbooks, and trade publications. We want to help others but wonder whether the exhaustion, frustration, and irritability we feel so much of the time is worth it. *What are we to do?*

Working in rural school districts, multiple urban schools, or several county skilled nursing facilities with teachers, psychologists, principals, occupational and physical therapists social workers, nurses, and other staff but, typically, with no other speech-language pathologist, we may feel marooned. We may find maintaining our sense of professional identity acquired as a graduate student difficult. To fit in, we may agree to perform duties, such as playground or lunchroom monitoring, we would refuse as inappropriate if another speech-language pathologist was present. We find altering our professional identity from the one we were taught to uphold brings additional stress. *What are we to do?*

3) *Recognizing our interconnectedness with those with whom we work.* We may misinterpret the responsibility we carry to help clients effectively communicate; identify, structure, and carry-out every-day tasks appropriately; and/or swallow safely. We may find it hard to draw upon the knowledge, experience and skills of colleagues and caregivers to help fashion meaningful, functional short-and long-term goals and address them because we believe relying on others to do our work could lead to a lack of respect for us and our profession. So, we decide to do the impossible, i.e., go it alone. We fail to recognize that soloing not only increases our already intense feeling of being burdened, contributes to our exhaustion, and heightens the probability of burning-out but also is improbable. Quantum mechanics and most

mystical traditions teach that each of us is embedded in a time-space matrix populated by all of which we are aware and much of which we are not with which we continually interact, knowingly and only dimly, if at all. We are not alone. To believe we can act alone is not only unrealistic it is unhelpful. *What are we to do?*

We Always Have a Choice

To effectively exercise our right to choose, we benefit from noting and evaluating the data we collect by listening carefully to our self-talk, recognizing that self-talk directs what we do and what we do not do and influences how we feel. Some self-talk is accurate and helpful. Some is false and misleading. Much of the unhelpful self-talk stems from conclusions we made early in life about who we are and what we can accomplish. By attending carefully to these silent messages we send ourselves, we can detect fear-based, self-defeating messages we may habitually send ourselves whenever we consider changing. Common ones include: *"It's too late; you should have started long ago." "This isn't for you!" "What will your friends think?"* and *"Don't rock the boat!"* Then we challenge them with our new-found knowledge of ourselves and the world around us (e.g., Katie, 2003; 2007). We can then, if need be, substitute accurate, affirming, and encouraging messages that keep us moving toward our goals for those that block our passage. The way to monitor self-talk is first to slow down. Slowing down enhances insight.

WAYS OF SLOWING DOWN

I walk more slowly than I have at other times during my adult life because that is what the limited range of motion of my right hip and knee requires. Hobbling a bit as I concentrate on walking safely, I often humorously visualize myself awkwardly illustrating Zen Master, Thich Nhat Hanh's instructive book, *Peace is Every Step* (Hanh, 1992). But, sometimes, when I am inclined to feel sorry for myself, I become embarrassed or angry if I believe neighbors or pedestrians think of me, a grey-haired, slightly stooped woman limping across my front porch, as flawed. That is when I instruct myself to stop *thinking of myself as flawed.* Whether they do or not, if I think that way, I will feel and act that way. And speculating about whether and how those around me may or may not be judging me interferes with appreciating what is, which is that by walking slowly, I notice more of what is about me than I did when I speed-walked. Recognizing that, I feel pleased with my present self. I automatically calm down and open up. I notice the corners of my mouth rise, forming a gentle, self-satisfied smile. And I respond this way more promptly the next time and relatively more so the time after that if I notice I am playing out that fantasy scenario of what others think of me as I walk about until it extinguishes.

Often I recall an earlier time when I could not walk at all because spinal polio forced me into relative inactivity. That was in the late '40's when I was five years old, months before our family, which did not own a phonograph, purchased a television set. Without any diversions, such as a radio, toys or books, or companionship, as I spent hour-after-hour laying on my back in bed practicing what was called "flat bed rest," I amused myself by being curious about the life I could see, hear, smell, taste, and touch. Einstein reportedly used his mind as his laboratory. I used mine as a playground where I imagined what was and could be. For instance, I would imagine faces taking form in the folds, creases, and recesses of the green-trimmed, white chenille curtains. I believed they had stories to tell, and I listened carefully to hear what they were. This curiosity has served me well when I slow down enough to release it, as I do in summer.

Summer is when our awareness of life expands once again. We notice life all around us. We see tomato, cucumber, and cup plants enlarging, flowering, and bearing fruit. Cement ants purposely parading down our front walk. White clouds stretching and reorganizing against a blazing blue sky. We hear the mourning doves' soulful song and auto horns blaring until owners return to turn them off. We notice power mowers and edgers used to tidy up neighbors' yards and enjoy the aromas their freshly cut grass gives off. We sense life more fully and move more slowly. We savor life's basics elements: The sun's warmth against our exposed skin, a towering silver maple's wisdom, a sparkling lake or vast ocean's demonstration of life's rhythms, a ladybug's faithfulness, and a grandchild's unfolding life. In summer, we simplify. We wear less clothing and move more freely. We live more by life's rhythms and less by the clock. We settle and observe. We slow down.

Slowing down to the pace of summer helped release me from the state of mental and physical constriction I often felt working 40-hour weeks in healthcare. There everyone's role seems to have been defined by management as essentially that of assembly line worker. Expected to repetitively contribute to the job of constructing someone's better life within a cold, grey world of ritualized sameness we, ironically, depleted our own. Working our way through daily schedule checks, staffings, paperwork, and rigidly timed meetings with patients leaves us feeling angry. We fantasize about securing another job in another place where we can apply our knowledge and skill with the care we wish to help people live better lives while enlarging our own. Then something arises to remind us of summer. A client improves dramatically. A colleague surprises us by bringing a cup of freshly brewed coffee to our desk. A caregiver looks relieved instead of anxious. We brighten and expand like a flower unfolding.

The reality, though, is that summer is but one of four seasons during the year. While it can be a glorious time to refresh our bodies and minds, we need not wait for it to recharge. We can fashion opportunities for rest and renewal throughout the entire year, each and every week. Most of us already care for our bodies. We attend to what and how we eat. We are careful to maintain our hydration. We exercise. We may even practice *hatha yoga* at studios and at home to become more flexible. And we appreciate the need to sleep well and enough. But we often overlook the necessity to steady, calm, and strengthen our minds. As Sakyong Mipham Rinpoche, Tibetan Buddhist Lama and best-selling author, advises, we need to care for our minds because they influence our every thought, feeling, and action

(Mipham, 2006). To calm and strengthen our minds, we cultivate patience and endurance. We can do that with a mind-care practice that includes meditation, personal journaling, and drawing and painting.

MEDITATION

Meditation can be a secular and non-secular practice and has been for centuries. So, too, can it be an individual and a group activity. The approach I describe here is basically non-secular and personal, though, at times, spontaneous prayer may infuse an experience if we are so disposed, and group meditation may strengthen individual practice. These approaches to mental quiet and expansiveness, as I have experienced them, lead to a helpful state of being where we can be a help rather than a hindrance (e.g., Wiegela, 1996) to ourselves and others, as long as we regularly undertake them.

The Genesis and Brief History of a Practice

For me, loath to fit more activity into already clogged workdays, the most accommodating way to practice slowing down initially was to embrace the Sabbath, sometimes defined as "*. . . an island in time*" (e.g., Heschel, 2005; Muller, 2000). As a Jew, I celebrated Sabbath Friday evening, when Sabbath begins, as a special *TGIF* event with a home-cooked meal shared leisurely with my daughter at the dining room table set with the good china. For years, we rediscovered ourselves and each other during those meals through unhurried conversation and loving communion with our two cats. Perhaps, because my intent was to establish a space in time where we could realign with one-another, I felt no pressure or strain preparing those meals. On the contrary, I almost reveled in the mental and physical activity. Later, when she moved away, I ate alone to reacquaint myself with my inner nature and to continue a refreshing practice. The following day, the Sabbath, I practiced wholeness with abandon. No matter what activities I might choose for a given Saturday, I included the opposites of solitude and solidarity. For many years, singing songs of worship together in the morning with a small group of congregants then sharing bread and wine together anchored the specialness of the day, the remainder of which I spent off-clock in quiet. By observing *havdalah*, a ceremonial rite marking the close of Sabbath and the beginning of the new week, seemingly grew an increasing longing to experience the sweetness and clarity of Sabbath throughout the week. Inhaling the fragrance of cloves rising from the freshly agitated spice box to remember the sweetness of Sabbath stirred a desire within me to cling to Sabbath-time and Sabbath-me. I wanted to remain the relaxed, curious, open, riding-the-wave Sabbath-self I was coming to savor and not morph into the automaton I resembled each work day.

Returning to a meditation practice begun years earlier, even when I thought I was too busy with single-parenting, and career-building to do one more thing, helped meet that desire.[2] When I foolishly told people I was meditating, they tried to discourage me. They thought I might "bliss-out." That was in the early-80's in fairly conservative Milwaukee, when those in my acquaintance considered meditation exotic and a free pass to cult membership. But I quietly persisted because I preferred the practice to the only alternatives I knew to calm down: Therapy and mood stabilizers. I believed meditation offered a truer path to wholeness than accommodating to another's plans for me and carried none of the short- and long-term risks ingesting pharmaceuticals could present someone who often experienced unwanted side-effects from medications. And, not incidentally, the financial cost of a meditation practice was negligible. Purchasing books, tapes, CD's, and DVD's to inform and support my practice involved a substantially inconsequential outlay compared to what I could be expected to pay for therapy and medication. And, with a few exceptions, I already owned the furniture and accoutrements with which I furnished my meditation space. The cymbal, incense, candle, and *tangka,* a Tibetan Buddhist iconic painting, that I purchased as specialty items collectively cost less than $130. Minus the tangka, the total cost was under $20.

As in the past, I found meditating, or sitting as it is often called, slowly rewarded me with a developing awareness of what I was experiencing internally and externally at a given moment and a growing perspective to distinguish the important from the unimportant. This brought occasional moments of calm that provided no small measure of relief from the anxiety I usually felt about whether I was doing enough and doing well enough. That does not mean my mind was still as I sat. On the contrary, it spun fantasies, recalled hurts, and envisioned catastrophes. My mind filled with thoughts and generated emotions the way it did when I drove. Whether I drove from home to the health foods store, transported my pet to the vet, traveled up north for a weekend, or toured the city with a friend or two, I recalled little of what I had seen as I drove. My mind was so busy creating and playing out *scenarios.* Meditation was no different the way I practiced it. I lit a white candle and, occasionally, a stick of incense, struck the cymbal, and settled into my chair. Almost immediately, my galloping mind dragged me here and there until, anxious or bored, I rose, invited the cymbal to ring once again, extinguished the candle flame, and left the room. I dutifully continued the practice once a day because by doing so I could console myself with the thought that, at least if I was not consistently content throughout the day, I was committing to becoming so to benefit myself and others, even if I could not know when and whether that might happen.

As I continued this practice, I learned more about the process by reading and listening to audio and video tapes and CD's. When I discovered mindfulness meditation, sometimes referred to as *vispassana* (e.g., Hanh, 2000; Kabat-Zinn, 2005; Kornfield, 1998), I knew that was the practice I had been seeking. To be more effective personally and professionally (e.g., Carroll, 2007), I knew I needed to know when and what I was seeing, hearing, feeling, tasting, and smelling as well as thinking each and every moment. I learned mindfulness meditation would help me train my mind to be more present more of the time, comparable to knowing where I was and what I was doing each moment I drove. And the practice could help me monitor my self-talk more consistently to detect and effectively deal with my core beliefs as they surfaced.

After a time of recognizing notable benefits, such as an increased ability to direct my mind rather than letting it bob up and down like a cork at sea, I realized I was refusing to accept thoughts and feelings I found disagreeable. I mentally swatted them away. They were as unwelcome as gnats flying at my face. Only pleasant thoughts and sensations for me, thank you! But after considering Pema Chödrön's teachings on *shenpa* (2003; 2005b), I knew I needed to change my view. I had studied psychology enough to know refusing to own and integrate personal dark and, perhaps, shameful qualities and characteristics breeds nasty consequences. They reappear more strongly with the potential to wreak havoc in our lives (e.g., Jung, 1997; 1976). Acknowledging that, I incorporated *shenpa* practice into my mindfulness practice (e.g., Silverman, 2005).

Another benefit I am realizing by meditating is *projecting* less (Please see Chapter 1). The combined mindfulness and *shenpa* practice increasingly opens me to life as it is, rather than life as I expect or want it to be. That reduces my tendency to displace my thoughts and feelings about circumstances and individuals by inappropriately ascribing them to others. For instance, I am now far less likely to relate to administrators as my parents and to friends as saviors. I, thankfully, am more likely to relate to them as individuals rather than as stand-in's for others with whom I have strong emotional attachments or desires with much more pleasant consequences for all of us. I am more present more of the time. *By being present*, I can experience life as a succulent fruit to be savored rather than as a fast food meal to slam into my mouth then quickly forget until I stand on the bathroom scale. *By being present*, I can readily recall what I experience in detail rather than straining to recapture uncertain slivers of life the way I work at recalling dreams. *By being present*, I can anchor myself to relate effectively in both the short- and long-run, rather than floating through life like a wispy, gossamer-like dream-walker whose effectiveness in this realm can be quite limited. *By being present*, I can discover who I am and help others do the same. And, *By being present*, patience becomes a more natural response.

Developing A Work-Related Personal Practice

While the goal of my meditation is simply to be present to thoughts, emotions, and sensations as they reveal themselves and to gently release them as I do, I am relating more effectively because I am listening more sensitively (e.g., Shafir, 2000). That, of itself enhances our work and our life. As we continue to meditate, we become more skillful because we are more present more of the time. We increasingly relate to clients, caregivers, students, colleagues, and administrators as who and what they are and less as projections of our own beliefs, thoughts, and feelings and, consequently, experience more satisfaction and less annoyance. We are happier. And we are more content because we are learning to appreciate *it is not all up to us*. We see our place in the change process and recognize the limits within which we work. Our beliefs and practices help prove the adage that when we do well for ourselves, we do well for others. Just like the mother who makes her well-being a priority in order to parent more effectively, we practice first and foremost for our own sakes.

Sitting and Moving. I meditated while working in an outpatient rehabilitation facility in the late 80's. Occasionally, during so-called lunch breaks and following the last scheduled appointment for the day, I placed my attention on my breath or on the flowers in the poster of a Van Gogh painting hanging above my desk. When I detected a thought, whether interesting, anxiety-arousing, or neutral, I immediately and gently released it to return to observing my in-breath's and my out-breath's or the structure and coloring of a particular flower or cluster of flowers. I meditated this way for 10 minutes or so. And for a considerable time afterward, I felt centered and peaceful. I do not think anyone realized I was meditating. No gongs rang out; no incense perfumed the air; and no chanting pulsed through the office and adjacent treatment corridor to signal I was. But I became more relaxed and happy. And I think those delightful energies may have radiated from me and may have been gratefully noticed.

I was working in what I considered a conservative region. Now it may be possible to openly meditate at work alone or with co-workers, since businesses and organizations are increasingly making wellness an on-site priority through healthier food choices offered in the cafeteria and vending machines, massage breaks, and the outfitted physical exercise areas where visualization and/or meditation also may be practiced. But, even in seemingly conservative surroundings, meditation can be practiced without fanfare to achieve a healthier environment for ourselves and others.

Although I was unaware of the practice of walking meditation (e.g., Nguyen and Hahn, 2006; Hahn, 1985) then, I often enjoyed walking alone for 10-15 minutes during our 30-minute lunch breaks. Free of the expectation to direct, tend to, or amuse another, those few minutes provided opportunity for real refreshment. As I trod from the Center at a modest pace, I allowed thoughts seeming to weigh me down to slip away like chiffon scarves riding the wind. Within a few minutes, relieved of much anxiety and resentment, my interested attention gravitated to what I could see, hear, smell, and feel. I noticed the trees lining the walk, the tall and short buildings, the sky, vehicles entering and leaving surface lots and parking structures. I heard flags snapping in the strong winds blowing through the open areas. I smelled organic aromas of mud, decay, and humidity. And the alternating rhythms of my arms and legs felt delightful. My breathing deepened. On the return portion of the walk, I was centered within my body, not as I had been at the start when, like James Joyce's character in the Dubliners, Mr. Duffy, I *"lived a short distance from my body."* And I usually remained centered most of the afternoon. Although I preferred solitary outings, I discovered walking with one or more individuals also could be centering, *if* all silently concentrate on the fullness of each present moment.

As we personally experience benefits from meditation, especially heightened concentration (e.g. Kabat-Zinn, 2005), we may come to believe clients with attending problems also may benefit from the cultivating their own practice. We may wish, for example, to inform parents of children we treat who have difficulty attending that children who meditate increase their ability to concentrate (e.g., Fontana and Slack, 1998; Rozman, 2002) and suggest to adults with stuttering problems that meditation may increase the ability to be present (e.g., Silverman, 2003d; 2005). But, unless we are teachers of meditation, we should make referrals to those who are and refrain from doing so as an element of the therapy we provide.

PERSONAL JOURNALING

Personal journaling, sometimes equated with keeping a diary, can help us reach deeply inward to uncover motives, feelings, and the basis for them. Individuals in the arts, sciences, and politics have long appreciated this tool as an accessible and private means to identify and extract previously unrecognized or cursorily acknowledged personal truths for study, reflection, and growth. For example, Alice Walker, Buckminster Fuller, John Adams, Harry Truman, May Sarton, Mary Chestnut, and others we may know have been or are dedicated journal keepers. Journaling relies on solitude, honesty, and perseverance to provide worthwhile results. The more we quietly probe, then reflect upon, our words and actions, deeds and misdeeds, and times of inaction, the more we become alert to our inner voice, which reminds us of who we are and what we need to do. As we read what we write about our experience, we realize, that by thoughtful writing, we are better able to discern our truth than we are when we speak or, even, when we think. There is something illuminating and palpable about our newly discovered sensibilities expressed as words we see. We can not blink them away. There they are. And there they stay, even when we stuff the pages on which they sit into a desk drawer, slam shut the book that contains them, or close the program in the computer where they reside. We have seen them, and we will not soon forget them, unlike words we can speak casually or thoughts that drift away. The words we write reflect what we have found to be true. This purposeful, thoughtful writing resembles the cutting and faceting of a rough diamond to release its beauty and value. Writing such as this helps us shine.

The chief difficulties I have encountered journaling stem from my relatively slow and often undecipherable handwriting and from a seeming lack of time to dig deeply into my psyche. Using a keyboard easily overcame the first obstacle because I can type almost as quickly as I can think in words and, then, I can actually read what I write. Finding time to journal was more challenging. Like everyone, my time is limited. To do all that I need and want on a daily basis usually requires more time and energy than I think I have. But thoughtful prioritizing provides time to journal when I want to, which is not when I am writing almost daily for publication. That is when I rely on other methods of self-knowledge to deepen my acquaintance with myself.

Asking and Answering "Why?"

My primary journaling method has been *Asking and Answering "Why"* (Please see Chapter 1) to identify core beliefs. Briefly, the process begins by selecting a recent unsettling experience to better understand why I feel as I feel and/or did what my action or inaction was that provoked the feeling. Then I describe the circumstance in writing, i.e., note those present, their role, and the physical surroundings including time of day, and record my feelings and/or actions as the event unfolded. Responding to the freshly written account, I write an answer to the question: *"Why did I feel that/act that way?"* Studying the answer leads to asking and writing an answer to *"Why did I think that?"* which I again ask after I answer, then repeat the process until I reach bedrock. There I discover the core belief that led to my discomfort and the actions I now regret. I know I have reached that critical place, that core belief, when my body-mind, upon recognizing it, relaxes instantly as if emitting a huge sigh.

After the initial feeling of warm relief from learning from analyzing a core belief what I can do to change my life for the better, dark feelings typically flooded my being when I began the practice. Those feelings of regret could enlarge quickly and create multiple aftershocks of embarrassment and shame. To forestall becoming stuck in those emotions that, if I let them, could lead to depression, I immediately relate to myself with kindness. I recall the affirming words of the poet and author Maya Angelou, who, said, *"When we know better, we do better."* I remember how less well I understood myself, others, and the world around me when I adopted that belief than I do now. I recognize my growth and my commitment to growth, and I celebrate that. I acknowledge there is no shame in admitting the need for change. On the contrary, there is great satisfaction in recognizing I am committed to being my best and doing my best. I make amends as appropriate and continue on.

That is how I proceed now. But, before I learned to look at life's challenges this way, I avoided core belief excavation. I did not want to fuel the despair I knew would envelope me by discovering evidence my family may have seen me correctly when they derisively called me "The Big Dummy." The effort required to detect what most likely would be a faulty core belief was easier to avoid than to undertake, even though I wanted to know myself better and do better, if doing the work might confirm I was "The Big Dummy." It was *shenpa* practice (e.g., Chödrön, 2005b: 2003; Silverman, 2005), more than any other influence, which emboldened me to calmly and steadfastly slide past that fear to proceed with the examination of my thoughts and behaviors. The central feature of the practice, as I understand it, is to remain with, rather than run from, uncomfortable thoughts, feelings, and emotions as they arise, change, and finally depart. By staying with and observing my fear or dislike until it naturally dissolves, I come to recognize some of the strength and courage I possess. That awareness helps offset the misplaced censure I prematurely applied to myself for having formed an unhelpful core belief. And that encourages me to continue the task as necessary and to do so with appreciation rather than dread. I now applaud my increasing strength and confidence to perform the work (Silverman, 2009), and I appreciate and admire Young Ellen-Marie for processing the limited information she had using an immature cognitive apparatus to discern how to grow, thrive, and contribute in, what, for her, was an extremely chaotic and hostile world.

Journaling Gratitude

Within the time span I encountered *shenpa* practice, I fortunately discovered another helpful approach to help me face and process unpleasant facets of myself. That was to summon feelings of gratitude (Boorstein, 2005). This practice balances *Asking and Answering "Why?"* Even though I desire self-knowledge, my ego tempts me to lay down that practice to avoid the shame and embarrassment I feel when I discover how I have thought and behaved to hurt myself and others. That is when examining a gift of the day becomes a gift of itself. Journaling about an unmerited gift reminds me I am essentially worthwhile despite needing work. Aren't we all?

When I contemplate the loyalty and patience of my animal companion, Hansom, who quietly waits for my attention while I write for hours; the red berries of the Hawthorne tree in my front yard feeding a small flock of cedar waxwings; the warm smile of a clerk at the deli department of a natural foods store as I stroll by; and the reliable service of the gas furnace warming the house during cold that can kill, I remember life is good. Not perfect, but good. Hansom barks incessantly as I place an order for lunch at the drive-through almost obliterating my request; the cedar waxwings excrete remnants of the berries onto the concrete walkway below; the deli clerk may be more interested in me making a purchase than the well-being of my psyche; and the almost constant running of my home furnace sends figurative dollar bills billowing out my chimney like a smoke plume rising from an erupting volcano. Choosing to bask in the feelings that arise within me as I recognize the goodness around me, I can more readily incorporate the recognition I, too, am not perfect but good. Feeling gratitude helps me think bigger.

I use a straight-forward journaling process to record feelings of gratitude at least once per week. The process I have found helpful involves:

A) *Selecting an experience that elicits feelings of gratitude that day.* I select the one that was most surprising, heartwarming, unfamiliar, and/or portends the most far-reaching consequences.

B) *Describing it.* I detail who or what was present, what occurred, where it occurred, what attracted me to the event, how it affects my beliefs of what is important, and how I plan live from then on

C) *Savoring the feeling of gratitude.* I quietly enjoy the feeling of warmth radiating from my abdomen, chest, throat, face and down my limbs and the ease and vastness of my mind as I write and afterward. I feel gratitude for the openness that contrasts so markedly with the cold, prickly feelings associated with the tightness I feel in my body and mind when I am hurried, anxious, and/or angry, if I actually attend to them then.

And

D) *Releasing it.* By letting go I re-align myself with an enlarged notion of reality in which I feel free to live with greater comfort and awareness of what life brings, i.e., gifts and challenges both, which, I'm beginning to believe, are one and the same.

I experimented with a third journaling method, The Progoff Intensive Journal® Program (Progoff,1983) for encounters with my subconscious mind. This detailed method experienced in a three-day introductory workshop helped identify and clarify motivations and patterns of thought and conduct in several areas of life, but I found it difficult to use without an instructor. So, I have settled on alternating between the methods of *Asking and Answering "Why?"* and *Expressing Gratitude.* Combining these two approaches, I experience islands in time in which, drawn to the center of my being, I find rest, healing, and encouragement and direction to continue.

DRAWING AND PAINTING

Many contemplative-type activities, in addition to mindfulness meditation and personal journaling, offer sure, safe opportunities to slow down. For instance, processing film or digital photographic images, writing poetry, creating and cultivating a garden, knitting, and, even, staring at a lava lamp can engage us completely enough to help us release for a while worries, fears, and anxieties to refresh and remember it is possible to be this way. Among such activities, drawing and painting remain my favorites. Grasping a pencil or a conté crayon to create a recognizable likeness of an object, person, or scene or mixing paints to apply to paper or canvas to produce a still life, portrait, or landscape invites me to direct, pleasurable, wordless experience that is incomparable.

When I draw or paint, I feel connected to who I am, a distinctly different experience from the feeling I experience behaving as a programmed robot when I focus on doing what it takes to consider myself successful. And that is why, when I was 37, I returned to drawing and painting to reclaim my life. I was startled into taking that action after I first envisioned myself for one brief, unpleasant moment as a salami being sliced into pieces, thick and thin, each eagerly grabbed and taken away by many hands. That image told me what I knew. I was disappearing. I had felt that way for some time. Leading a ferociously active life for years as a university professor, wife and mother and graduate and post-graduate student before then, I was spent psychically. The only time I allotted myself was when I rode my exercise bicycle, walked, or meditated. Meditating helped me settle down and bring a sense of calm and perspective to daily life. And, at this particular juncture, medi-tating provided the time and space to notice an insistent, surprising desire poking around the edges of my being: I ached to paint. The timing of this message was exquisite. I had received academic tenure the previous year, the prized imprimatur denoting professional respectability and responsibility, and, with it, the promise of economic security. This hap-penstance freed me to do or not do as I wished professionally, short of breaking the law, of course. And, so, I became a Sunday painter. Spending 1-2 hours alone Sunday after Sunday at my easel in a wordless world of subject, light, paint, turpentine, brushes, and canvas attending to line, edge, shadow, space, hue, and tint moment-by-moment began the enduring process of resuscitating the person I was. Creating images that reflected back to me what I thought and felt to be contemplated and incorporated, infused my being with a sense of self that enlarged in every respect. I stopped shrinking.

Realism

A painting teacher I knew instructed her class, *"Learning to draw is learning to see."* I have found that is so. And I have found that it is done by entering into a wordless space. To realistically capture a still life, scene, or visage, we apply what Alfred Korzybski (1955), founder of General Semantics, taught, *"The word is not the thing."* Words, those slippery tools of convention, filter our reality. They channel our perceptions. Only when we relate to the subject of our drawing or painting through what we actually see, i.e., angles, propor-tions, placements, shadows, lines, edges, filled and unfilled spaces, hues, tints, light, dark, and, what Betty Edwards (2001), teacher of realistic drawing techniques to adults who believe they can not draw, slyly refers to as the *thingness of the thing,* rather than through concepts encapsulated by words, such as *tree, old woman, baby, chair,* or *dance,* can we create realistic representations of our subjects. By abandoning labels, those short-cuts to engage-ment, to wordlessly and directly approach our chosen subject, the life we observe and the life within us interact in an uncharacteristically vivid manner that can lead to a recogniz-able representation. This may sound mystical or far-fetched if you have not experienced this. But it is possible to readily do so.

Drawing From Two Different Mind-Sets. Betty Edward (2001) refers to right-brain draw-ing and left brain drawing in the book she authored, *Drawing on the Right Side of the Brain.* The book includes references to her doctoral dissertation detailing the two different visual perceptual modes associated with our two cerebral hemispheres and exercises she developed to teac*h* untrained adults to draw realistically relying on the perceptual qualities of the right hemispheres. Examples she provides portray dramatic differences in student draw-ings from their first class to their final one, which may only be several days later.

You might be able to experience a taste of what she ably teaches by completing the fol-lowing task adopted from one of her signature exercises. If you do not, do not discount her method. She presents several exercises leading up to this one and provides more guidance than I do. I strongly encourage you go acquaint yourself with her clear, capable, and illuminating teaching methods.

First, obtain a photograph of a face you would like to draw. While working from life provides a surer means of communing with a subject to produce a representative portrait, dealing effectively with changing light where we draw might be too challenging for beginners. So place the photograph where you can readily see it in its entirety. Then draw the image on a clean, unlined sheet of paper at least 8.5" by 11.0" using a Number 2 pencil. Include all the detail you see. Put the drawing aside.

On the following day, make a second drawing of the photograph. Again, use a Number 2 pencil, and make your drawing on an 8.5" by 11.0" sheet of clean, unlined paper. *But, this time, turn the photograph upside-down.* Draw the inverted image exactly as you see it. Start at the top and move straight down the page until you have finished copying the image. Include all the detail you see. When you finish, flip it so it appears like the photograph. Compare the two drawings. If the experiment worked, the drawing of the upside-down photograph resembled more closely the image, since its unorthodox rendering disrupted our tendency to label what we believe we know from past experience, i.e., a human face based on the labels/concepts we have stored of eyes, nose, mouth, and so forth. Instead, the inverted/unfamiliar image for which we have few, if any labels, leads us to draw what we actually see before us.

That is why we put aside the literal meaning of Gertrude Stein's dictum that *". . . a rose is a rose is a rose. . ."* if we wish to live and work well. We recognize and appreciate individual characteristics of different roses and rosebuds, of different country scenes, and of different green bell peppers to faithfully portray our chosen subject as distinct, even as we quietly acknowledge its kinship with other roses, other pastoral landscapes, and other green bell peppers. And, as we relate deeply enough to our subjects to discover their singularities, we discover to our surprise and delight, we are deeply enriched because our sense of ourselves and our world has enlarged somewhat and, with that, our effectiveness as clinicians, researchers, and teachers. In contrast, our effectiveness shrinks when we come to believe "an aphasic is an aphasic," "a dysphagic is a dysphagic" and so forth, with no disrespect to Ms. Stein intended.

Drawing and painting slow us down, help us see, and foster the patience required to know and understand (e.g., Churchill, 1950). Participating in these activities, we stretch our consciousness by interacting more closely with *what actually is* rather than what *we think is*. And, later, if we chose to study our work by reflecting on the subject matter we selected, the materials we used, and the techniques we applied, previously submerged concerns and conflicts, fears and apprehensions, and growth and possibilities of growth may begin to reveal themselves. Acknowledging these helps ready us to continue our passage toward increasing self-awareness (e.g., Malchiodi, 2002; Silverman, 2008b). Drawing and painting provide tangible souvenirs of our life's passages to serve as chronology, maps to the future, gifts to share as we wish, and, not least, a serviceable metaphor for our approach to clinical work.

CODA

This is my story, the intersection of my life and work. I hope you will share yours. *Kabbalists* believe our individual stories highlight teachings of the *Torah,* or Jewish scriptures (Gafni, 2004). They call on us to claim then share our stories as the gifts each of us brings into this world. Holding back such a gift can be equated, on a primitive level, to baking chocolate, tofu, soy nut butter brownies to sweeten a staff meeting then choosing not bring them for fear of rejection. We may believe that some colleagues might consider us odd if they learn we baked with tofu and soy nut butter, some may criticize us for offering a processed carbohydrate confection rather than fresh fruit and vegetables, some may criticize us for bringing an unsolicited snack, which they consider an attempt to elevate our personal standing within the group, and so on. Each concern may be realistic and cause for ill-will, but they are not the only possible responses. Some may appreciate the opportunity to re-fuel by eating our protein-laden brownies. They may be the majority, or they may not. It doesn't matter. If we know some are hungry, and we can feed them, then why should we hold back? And so it is with our work-related learning. If we know colleagues seek new ideas, and we have discovered some time-tested ones, why should we hold back?

Had I not written *Mind Matters*, I would feel a nagging sense of guilt. Not sharing information with colleagues that can bring desired change more readily to them and their clients feels strangely selfish. Perhaps, what I have to say will be readily, even eagerly embraced or, perhaps, not. Maybe what I have written will inspire only one person. I have no guarantee I will be heard, that my message will be accepted or, even, received, but I feel I have done my job by communicating what I have learned about doing the work. Just as many older adults learn by sharing their personal stories with their children and grandchildren that a life that is shared is a life well-lived, so it is with a career.

APPENDIX A:

Creating Conditions for Change[1]

This paper, presented at the 10th Annual International Stuttering Awareness Day (ISAD) Online Conference, October, 2007, presents an overview of what is involved when working for desired, personal change. A threaded discussion consisting of comments and questions made to the paper and responses to them is available at http://cahn.mnsu.edu/10silverman. Since the core theme of Mind Matters involves the management of desired, personal change, I decided to make this paper available within the context of this book.

---

[1]© 2007 by Ellen-Marie Silverman

CREATING CONDITIONS FOR CHANGE

I am grateful to once again participate in this special forum. I know of no other conference about stuttering so accessible with more potential to provide genuine assistance than this one. So, "Thank You, Judy Kuster!" for sharing yet another burst of your inspiration and networking talent to prepare and present this helpful vehicle. And "Welcome!" to you, Dear Reader. I hope you will find something helpful in the thoughts I share about *Change*, something we all long for, dread, and deal with daily in one way or another. After 43 years of working with this process as a professional and more than that as an individual, I find I am just beginning to understand what is involved. And I am impressed by the courage and patience required.

Those of us who seek to change the way we communicate or to help someone else do that are the intended audience. What binds us together in common cause is the challenge to manage change in a manner that is liberating. I know for sure that relating well to change bolsters the process and that not doing so causes it to falter, even implode. What follows stems from my experience of what is necessary, what is helpful, and what is involved.

DEATH, TAXES, AND CHANGE

Wherever and whenever we are born and into what circumstance, among the basic elements of life we share are these: We die. We pay taxes. And we deal with change. Since we arrived in this world fresh from our mother's body, we have changed. Our bodies changed. They grew longer, wider, thicker. They grew whiskers. They grew bald. Our interests changed. No longer amused by lying on our back and sucking our toes, we rolled over and crawled. We listened to stories and songs, then wrote them. We longed to become an astrophysicist until we discovered *croissants* and fancied becoming a *chefs de cuisine*. Our thoughts about ourselves changed, too, from rapt attention during infancy to anxious assessment during childhood and beyond as we learned to compare our features, skills, and experiences with others and began wondering, *"Am I Good Enough?"* And, quite often, from then on, we thought we were not. We were too tall, too thin, too quiet, too awkward, too dumb, too poor, and so on. We wanted to fit in, maybe *"WOW"* our friends. We wanted to change.

Sometimes we did not know we needed to change, but our parents did. They may have decided we needed to stop stuttering, which, often, we did not know we were doing until they, or a relative, or the parent of a friend, or, maybe, a neighbor across the hall, or a classroom teacher said something to us such as, *"That was smooth. Cool!"* *"Slow down!"* *"Easy!"* We were quick to pick up we had to talk better to please those powerful people. We needed to change.

EXPERIENCES LAST

> *"Before you ask someone to change the world, make sure they like it*
>
> *the way it is."*
>
> - - - Vin Diesel, actor

I sometimes think there is nothing as durable as childhood experiences. They color our lives as they shape them. The murky interaction of our individual temperaments with our early experience as interpreted by our maturing cognitive apparatus establishes what we come to believe as true about ourselves, others, and the world (e.g., Chess and Thomas, 2005) and sets the stage for how we think, feel, and act from then on (e.g., Steiner, 1994) unless and until we recreate our individual cosmology. As a personal example, nothing influenced me more than my mother's death when I was three and one-half.

These are the basic facts: Late at night, the first day home from the hospital after delivering my sister *via* c-section, my mother began retching. The unfamiliar sounds first awakened then frightened me. I put on my slippers and ran into my parents' bedroom just across the hall. When I entered, I saw my mother lying on the far side of the double bed on her right side, her right arm cradling a white coated bucket. She and I were the only ones there. She lifted her head and held me with her eyes. They seemed larger than ever. Fear and love radiating from them held me in silence. She did not speak.

I was terrified. I had never seen my mother, my protector, weak and helpless. She resumed retching. My terror increased as I helplessly watched her body convulse and heard, once again, those wrenching sounds.

More than anything, I wanted her to stop. I wanted her to be herself. Not knowing what else to do, I jumped up and down, up and down, shouting, *"Shut-up. Shut-up."* Almost immediately, my father appeared. He quickly and tenderly carried me from their bedroom. Within moments, he prepared a place for us to sleep together on the living room floor, a few feet from their bedroom door. Early the next morning, he went in to check on her. Then the awful screaming began. She was dead. She had died from a hemorrhagic stroke while we slept.

These are my three and one-half year-old self's interpretations of those facts:

Words kill. I killed my mother with my words. I am a bad person. I am alone. I do not deserve to be loved ever again.

This is what I told myself and no one else at the time. And that is what I repeated to myself every now and again for many years thereafter whenever I experienced something that reminded me of that original experience. For instance, when I was 10 and in the fifth grade, our beloved principal, who looked and walked like a gracefully aging *prima* ballerina, uncharacteristically visited our class. She came to scold us. She warned us that no one was ever to say to anyone else the worst words that could be said. The words she banned in the classroom and forbade on the school yard were *Shut-up!* Shocked, I immediately flashed back to the night I shouted those very same words at my mother then never saw her again.

I heard our principal say more, but I did not listen to her words. I was acknowledging to myself I was as bad as I thought. I was deeply ashamed. I felt I was sinking.

Eventually, I no longer remembered the words of my interpretations. But they already had set patterns of perception and behavior into motion that colored my entire life until I recalled them several decades later and challenged them kindly but firmly using my adult knowledge and experience.

Nevertheless, the beliefs they fostered that I was horrid and unworthy of love and that spoken words can kill still emit silent sprouts that I continue to toil at uprooting.

This particular example may be unique, but the tendency to interpret experience is not. It is common-place for all of us, children and adults. And, in fact, it is our interpretation of what we experience that affects us more so than the experience itself (e.g., Chess and Thomas, 2005; Steiner, 1994). For children, interpretations are especially noteworthy. First, because children lack the knowledge, experience, and capacity to draw the measured conclusions an adult might. And Secondly, the conclusions children draw have far-reaching consequences for how they live their lives from then on. We need to take this into account when we arrange to have a child tested or enrolled in speech therapy. Children's generally unspoken interpretations of why they are having new experiences and what those experiences mean, what they have to do be successful in them, and how they need to be to be accepted and, thereby, survive all need to be seriously considered. While we may never exactly know their interpretations of testing or therapy experiences, we can be certain they are making them, e.g., *Jason's Secret* (Silverman, 2001). Therefore, to paraphrase Vin Diesel, the actor quoted at the start of this section,

Before we ask children to change,

Let's be sure to first teach them to love themselves just as they are.

If we do that, their self-worth will be based on who they are, not on what they do, how they do it, or what they have, and they will have a good chance to live genuinely happy, satisfying lives. *If we teach them to love themselves*, they will seek the best for themselves and strive to have it. *If we teach them to love themselves,* they will do all that is necessary to materialize the change they want, if and when they decide to change how they look, act, or think. And *If we teach them to love themselves,* they can love.

PENTIMENTO

" . . . pentimento . . . a change of mind . . . a way of seeing and then seeing again."

- - - Lillian Hellman, Playwright, Author (1973)

At some point in our lives, we may come to feel stuck. We find that although we have changed our jobs we experience the same relationships with co-workers and supervisors we detested before. We notice that even when we align with new partners we experience the same unpleasant "push-pull" relationship we had with so many others before. We join a different faith community only feeling the need to fend off fellow worshippers behaving as annoyingly intrusive as the ones in the faith community we left behind. And, despairingly, we may observe that our stuttering problem is no better or worse than it was years earlier despite our fervent desire and, occasional, intense efforts to rid ourselves of it. If we want to change what we experience, we come to realize, we will have to change at the most basic level.

During my undergraduate clinical training in stuttering problems, I encountered a woman with a stuttering problem who had achieved a certain notoriety at our university speech clinic. She, someone in her mid-30's who worked as a secretary in a large firm, had learned each of Van Riper's various stuttering control techniques. She would proudly demonstrate her mastery of their mechanics behind closed doors in treatment but nowhere else because, in her words, *"They don't feel natural."* Marcy, not her real name, showed that changing the mechanics of speech is not synonymous with personal change, although it can certainly lead to that.

Those of us with stuttering problems come to know changing how we talk then changing how we communicate can change our lives. And, as paradoxical as it first may seem, we sometimes choose to keep our lives just as they are even though doing so means continuing to experience the fear, shame, and embarrassment of stuttering we detest because, fundamentally, we are comfortable (e.g., Myss, 1998). Although our lives, like everyone else's, are not always pleasant, they are fairly predictable. We've got them under control, at least most of the time. And that is what so many of us crave, especially in these uncertain times. We want to know where we will be having breakfast today, what we'll be doing Sunday morning, where we will shop Friday after work, when we will be vacationing, and so on. If we change how we communicate, we will change how we live. We may change jobs. We may change relationships. We may change locales. The winds of change may transport us to a very different life gradually or swiftly. We can not be sure. That is why change requires courage and endurance, the courage to let go of the past to move into an uncertain future along an unknown path and the commitment to take the ride as far as it goes for as long as it takes. As long as we prefer the comfort of the known over the risk of the unknown, we will not sincerely work for the change we say we would like to have.

We will change, nevertheless. That is inevitable. We will become both more and less like we currently are. Our habits will grow stronger until our physical and, perhaps, our mental capacities will grow weaker. Our circumstances will change. Friends and loved ones will move away. Some will die. New people will become important. Work outside the home will change or end. We may develop hobbies that engage us. Nothing about us will stay the same except, perhaps, for a while, our perceptions of how our life is and should be. Until we change them, we will fundamentally live as we have until the very end (e.g., Byrne, 2006; Chess and Thomas, 2005; Hellman, 1973; Myss, 1998; Silverman, 2006; Steiner, 1994). Remember:

> *"A foolish consistency is the hob-goblin of little minds. . ."*

> - - - Ralph Waldo Emerson

> *Self-Reliance in Essays, Second Series (1847)*

REFERECES

Byrne, R, Ed. (2006). <u>The Secret</u>. New York: Atria Books.

Chess, S. and Thomas, A., (2005). <u>Temperament in Clinical Practice</u>.

New York: The Guilford Press.

Hellman, L. (1973). <u>Pentimento</u>. Boston: Little, Brown, and Company.

Myss, C. (1998). <u>Why People Don't Heal and How They Can</u>. New York:

Three Rivers Press.

Silverman, E.-M. (2006). Mind Matters. Presented at the 9th Annual International

ISAD Online Conference, October.

Silverman, E.-M., (2001). <u>Jason's Secret</u>. Indianapolis: 1st Books.

Steiner, C. (1994). <u>Scripts People Live</u>. New York: Grove/Atlantic Press.

APPENDIX B

Learning to Sit[1]

The motivation and experimentation that evolved into my current meditation practice has taught me, after 20 years, to meditate, not just "sit." The practice, a co-mingling of shenpa practice (Silverman, 2005) and mindfulness meditation (Silverman, 2003d) brings calm, clarity, and joy into my daily life and helps me effectively address a long-seated stuttering problem. The practice teaches me to attend closely to my seemingly constant self-talk to help implement and stabilize constructive, alternative responses to feelings of helplessness, anxiety, and embarrassment when I stutter.

LEARNING TO SIT

For a long time, I have not been very good at sitting, a common vernacular for meditating. Whether or not I meditated when I sat the past three and one-half decades was questionable. Except for my introduction to meditation, when for a few weeks I doggedly repeated a mantra assigned by a Transcendental Meditation instructor and the several occasions I participated in guided visualizations after that, I variously and passively occupied the seat of a green upholstered chair in which I fed my infant daughter years earlier, a high-back teak dining room chair with a cushioned, wide black vinyl seat, or a black shovel seat Boston Rocker purchased as a parenting tool while mostly lost in thought yet certain I was meditating.

My instruction about assuming a sitting position simply had been: Sit in a chair. Place both feet flat on the floor. Rest your hands on your thighs, palms down. So that is what I did for the first few weeks until I felt the need to change my hand position. Years later, without forethought, I modified their position once again. Recently, I altered their position a third time to hands on thighs palms up, thumb tips gently pressing tips of middle fingers. I have since learned this hand *mudra*, the *shuni mudra,* facilitates patience. Very apt.

Settled in the chair *du jour,* I almost immediately gave my thoughts free-rein, and they carried me here and there and back, a familiar experience and, as familiar, vaguely comforting. Planning. Wishing. Worrying. Plotting. Ruing. That was what I did when I sat. I learned to amuse myself with thought as a child. Seemingly at whim, my stepmother forced me to sit without company or entertainment for hours on end on my bedroom chair, a devilishly ironic birthday present from her when I turned 10. I sat stiffly, feet planted on the floral patterned linoleum floor in that green chintz cushioned chair with its dainty pleated skirt while gripping the rounded ends of its pine arms. Immersing myself deeply in dark thought was my reactive, angry, defensive response to the sitting alone bombarded by the stream of irritating, taunting sound rising from the living room. There my sister, stepmother, and father shared a raucous solidarity watching television shows after dinner. Their twisted combinations of consonants and vowels, vocal pitch and pause helped me fashion a perception of myself as outcast that guides me still. Much later, with some relief and gratitude, I realized theirs was a camaraderie from which I fortunately had been spared. So sitting immersed in thought was familiar. Nothing to fear. I decided to continue what I believed was meditating.

I took up sitting because I was desperate for relief from constriction in my life. Working to secure academic tenure while carrying almost sole responsibility for a difficult six-year-old daughter and dealing with an emotionally distant, soon to be ex-husband left me about to crumble. Because my childhood taught me to fear change I did not script, I initially rejected meditation as a means of relief, believing it to be a powerful catalyst for deep-seated change. But the acute need I felt to calm and balance my frantic mind paired with my distrust of "the talk cure" and serious apprehensions about the long-term effects of pharmacological intervention left sitting, the tool of my childhood limitation, the possible means to my liberation.

Years of sitting atop the run-away thought horse on occasional weekday afternoons to claim needed personal space, or so I thought, eventually helped lead me to *dharma* study. Twenty years after I first sat to meditate, now living alone with no one to care for but myself and refashioning my life, I was searching for practical guidance to live meaningfully second by second, day by day. I remembered a surprising gift from a staunch Methodist friend several years earlier, a book she received traveling in Hawaii. The slim volume presented key Buddhist teachings. From the outset, the content warmly engaged my mind and heart. I believed I had found the direction and alliance I had been seeking all my life. But unwilling to release myself from a conflicting, congenital affiliation with Judaism and unaware of the possibility of being a *Jew-Bhu*, I studied no further until my daughter unexpectedly declared Buddhist studies as one of her two undergraduate majors.

The time for me to study dharma seemed right. Borrowing the structure of my expiring *Torah* study, I began reading contemporary writings daily shortly after rising. Then I sat. Whether *Theravadan* or *Vajrayana* in perspective, the readings touched me deeply. I fell in love as I had earlier studying and practicing Judaism and Transactional Analysis. Each, by outlining a compelling perspective on personal responsibility and choice, functioned like forceps to extract fresh life from an out-grown world view, like revealing the child doll beneath the outermost ones in a set of nesting dolls. I felt giddy embracing the possibilities.

I also felt wretched. A helper by nature and profession, being blocked from directly helping others as I was accustomed led me to experience hopelessness. I had made a startlingly unwise career choice driven by spite that ejected me from a sphere of influence to place me in an unheralded position from which I could not retrace my steps. Contrasting what had been with the limitations I currently faced led me, for whom work was everything, to loneliness (e.g., Cacioppo and Patrick, 2008) and multiple dark days. My angst was not unlike that of my traumatically brain-injured adult patients who, after weathering weeks of treatment, realized they could not return to their life as it was. Not to the same schooling or employment. Not to the same relationships. Not to their dreams. All was forever changed. And all seemed less. I, at least, could live independently.

I held fast to my practice as I had earlier to *Torah* study. *Dharma* study became, as *Torah* study had before, the haven where I could experience the resonance of truth I had longed to hear. I came to understand by changing myself I would inevitably and genuinely create good ripples, if not directly in the ocean, then, in a tide pool that would, in its own way and time, release them to the sea. I realized my life was my work. Not career. Not family.

Not friends. But my life. I selected mindfulness as the means to acquaint me with my life to live it as it was. I dug in.

In the process, I read Pema Chödrön's paper on *shenpa*, habitual responses that draw us from the present to meet our need for comfort, in the March, 2003, issue of *Shambhala Sun*. She likened *shenpa* to scratching an itch and identified *shenpa* as both the itch and the scratching. After a page or so, I knew working with *shenpa* was what I had been seeking most of my life. As a speech pathologist and someone who has an intermittent stuttering problem, I believed reducing the *shenpa* of stuttering could help release me and others from its physical, emotional, and cognitive aspects. With this practical goal, I excitedly shifted the focus of my practice from mindfulness, as such, to working with *shenpa*. I became more focused, more interested in noting what I was thinking, feeling, and doing. Finally, I was beginning to meditate more of the time I sat and even when I was moving around.

I believe that for ultimate benefit I need to free myself of expectation and surrender to relate to what is as it is. I hope I learn that, as my exit from this life looms closer. Yet, without seeking to help myself and others find freedom from stuttering problems, I doubt I would be doing other than the drifting I have done the many previous years I sat. With that goal and the structure working on *shenpa* offers, I am experiencing increased awareness of life and how I respond to it. I am not just sitting. I am meditating.

APPENDIX C

HAPPILY EVER AFTER[1]

Like our clients, we occasionally quit programs designed to help us change something about ourselves to become happy because we fail to achieve the results we seek as comfortably and as quickly as we would like or because we fear we may actually change and no longer live the life we know. This paper, presented at the 11th Annual International Stuttering Awareness Day (ISAD) Online Conference, October, 2008, considers some of the dynamics involved when seeking change for happiness' sake that are as applicable to us as they are to those dealing with a stuttering problem. A threaded discussion of the paper consisting of comments and questions and my responses to them is available at http://cahn.mnsu.edu/11silverman as well as the paper itself.

---

[1] *© 2008 by Ellen-Marie Silverman*

HAPPILY EVER AFTER

Call me Hag or call me Crone. At 65, I've earned the tags. But I prefer the title Elder. I've lived a lot. I've learned a lot. And I feel responsible to pass on what little wisdom I've acquired. That's what elders do. So, allow me to me do some non-institutionalized *eldering* (Shacter-Shalomi, 1997) by sharing some hard-won knowledge about living happily ever after. But, first, a heartfelt *"Thank You!"* to Prof. Judy Kuster, Chair of this special forum for the 11th consecutive year, for offering the space to do this. *Kudos* to her once again for bringing so many together to inform and encourage each other about managing stuttering problems, our own or someone else's. And *"Welcome!"* to you, Dear Reader.

FEELING HAPPY

I'm more fluent than ever; I should feel happy.

* * * * *

I've been accepted to graduate school by my first choice; I should feel happy.

* * * * *

My child is participating in classroom discussions and making friends; I should feel happy.

* * * * *

BUT I DON'T!

Isn't that the way! We get what we want, and, for a while, we are happy. Then we discover what we received does not perfectly match what we expected. And, *Poof!* Anger, sadness, or fear replaces our happiness. Consider:

1) We stutter as fiercely and as much or more than ever days after an amazingly fluent weekend in a fluency workshop, and we crumble for a time. Although we soon resume passably fluent speech, we no longer feel confident interacting because a nagging doubt about whether we will ever be truly fluent drags us down.

2) When we arrive on campus as a new grad student, we discover that continuing grad students are closed and shun friendly contacts with new students. A sharp ache in the pit of our stomach quickly replaces the excitement we felt thinking about socializing with fellow students. We don't want to be part of such a cold culture, but, for financial reasons, we see no other choice but to stay

AND

3) Our child stutters as much as ever, sometimes more tensely, now that he is making presentations, participating in discussions, and playing with friends.

Our anxiety about whether therapy will work for him and whether we en-rolled him in the right program replaces the elation we felt when he began opening up.

We could discuss why it is that reverting from happy to sad in each instance is un-necessary, but I selected these examples for another purpose, i.e., to pose the question, *Can we experience lasting happiness?* I think many of us quietly ponder this possibility from time-to-time because we know the hope, indeed, the expectation that we can drives us to enter therapy, to apply to the best graduate programs, to carefully consider decisions for our children, and to make each and every choice count has not yet resulted in everlasting happiness. Sometimes we even may slip into despair, doubting that happiness is for us, concluding it is only for others. From personal experience, I know how easy it is to think this way. I grew up believing what fairy tales taught: If you thought good thoughts and did good deeds, someone or something would rescue you from your bitter situation to live "Happily Ever After." Some years ago, I realized just how strongly that belief affected me when, alone and deeply distressed about facing a series of troubling circumstances, I surprised myself by shouting out to the ether, *"I want my 'Happily Ever After!'"* Frustrated after decades of patterning my life after fairy tale heroines who received the gift of happi-ness everlasting while I did not, my roar was a bit like the Seinfield character Mr. Costanza, George's father, bellowing, *"Serenity Now!"* when he could not bear feeling undone one second longer. Examining the beliefs I held that lead to that startling reaction helped put me on The Path of Happiness, which I have determinedly traveled since. So, my response to the question, based on knowledge and personal experience, is a definite, *"Yes!"* We can conduct ourselves in a way to be genuinely happy (e.g., Kornfield, 2008: Seligman, 2004) most of the time. Here's how.

NOW OR NEVER

Be happy now! There is no need to wait until therapy fixes us, or we become a certified clinician, or our child no longer stutters. And most of us know it is futile to depend on a fairy godmother or handsome prince to *happify* us. So, if we wait until we and everything we care about are just as we wish, happiness will forever elude us. We will be one speech hesitancy, one clinical certification requirement, or one stuttering episode away. We do not have to live like that. We have the capacity to be happy right where we are no matter how dire the circumstance, not by relenting or settling but by altering our view, and we possess the power to do so once we realize that. For instance, centuries ago, British poet Richard Lovelace wrote from prison, *"Stone walls do not a prison make, nor iron bars a cage;"* and, last century, logotherapy founder, psychiatrist Viktor Frankl (2006) recounted that he survived Nazi concentration camp internment by embracing two thoughts which gave him happi-ness, rejoining his wife and completing a technical manuscript. Others, informed by their knowledge of sacred texts and personal experience, e.g., Tolle, (2005), Hanh (2004), and

Myss (1997), also assert it only is in the present where we can experience happiness. As Loretta La Roche (1995), humor therapist, reminds us, *"The past is history. The future is a mystery. Now is a gift. That's why it's called The Present."*

Pema Chödrön (2006) and other students of human happiness, including Tsultrim Allione (2008) and Martin Seligman (2004), teach us to create enduring happiness for ourselves that can accommodate life's up's and down's, including periods of grief and loneliness, by accepting both "agreeable and disagreeable" as they appear in our lives. For most, doing so initially is contrary to our more instinctive response of resisting what we do not want and doggedly chasing after what we think will remove or lessen our pain. But, by resisting our unpleasant thoughts, feelings, and sensations as we stutter and others' real and imagined negative responses as we do, many of us have layered our stuttering problems with throbbing complexity. As the late Wendell Johnson (1956) cautioned more than a half century ago, a stuttering problem is *". . . an anticipatory, apprehensive, hypertonic avoidance reaction. . . "* and, as such, thrives on resistance. In addition to feeding our stuttering problem, resistance delays our opportunity to learn from carefully studying how we think, act, and feel as we stutter to discern which mind-sets and behaviors we need to release and which to cultivate to speak with increasing ease and finesse. And, by welcoming, rather than resisting, stuttering, as paradoxical as such a choice seems until we do it, we gain enhanced self-esteem (Silverman, 2005).

It is hard to imagine anyone who dwells on what makes them unhappy about the way they speak and about themselves as a speaker benefiting much from speech therapy, unless and until they discover what also makes them happy about how they speak and themselves as speakers. As actor, writer, director, and producer Vin Diesel succinctly stated:

"Before you ask someone to save the world,

make sure they like it just the way it is."

Seeing ourselves broadly as we actually function, i.e., as partners, brothers, sisters, fathers, mothers, friends, colleagues, gardeners, community members, etc. demonstrating our individual strengths and weakness rather than through the tightly closed, smudged window of labels, such as female, Jew, Latina, senior citizen, stutterer, and, especially, PWS, (acronym for person who stutters), which diminish our perception of who we are and what we can do for ourselves and others is a good place to start. Therapy and self-help groups which anchor us in a larger, more realistic personal perspective than labels allow are likely to stimulate and support healing because such an orientation is apt to help us think well of ourselves (e.g, Hanh, 2004).

KINDNESS

When we think we deserve to be happy, we treat ourselves kindly. Many of us, after experiencing stuttering-related hurt, choose to be "nice" people. We appear agreeable and encouraging in public, but, in private, especially during our almost continuous self-talk, denigrate ourselves for failing to live up to our standards with associates, family, friends, and strangers because we stuttered or because we believed we squandered an opportunity to be helpful or for personal advancement through our fear of stuttering. This sort of self-abasement that can readily lead to unnecessary disengagement from others (e.g., Silverman, 2003; 2006) contributes to a mix of dreary and miserable feelings while strengthening stuttering-related avoidant behaviors (e.g., Allione, 2008). Like the legendary French chanteuse Edith Piaf, who lived so challenging a life that she died at 47 appearing years older, yet came to resonate with one of her signature songs, *"No. No Regrets!"* we, too, gain nothing useful by burdening ourselves with feelings of regret and blame. When we release self-recrimination for stuttering, perhaps, we can relate kindly to ourselves. That is when we will find more of the contentment we seek.

CAUTION

Treading a Path of Happiness is not easy. Far from it! Doing so requires commitment to change, i.e., embarking on a journey which can take us we know not where; willingness to take personal responsibility for our choices; and application of honesty and courage, as much as we can muster, moment-by-moment. Some spiritual teachers (e.g., Gimian, 2008, p. 76) advise students, *"It is better not to begin such a journey, but, if you begin, you should go all the way to the destination."* I believe it is more difficult to suffer without knowing a way out than to face unknown challenges. So, I have chosen to walk a path rather than wander in the wilderness. For now, that brings enough reward.

REFERENCES

Written

Allione, T., (2008). <u>Feeding Your Demons</u>. <u>Ancient Wisdom for Solving Inner</u>

    <u>Conflict</u>. New York: Little, Brown and Company.

Frankl, V., (2006). <u>Man's Search for Meaning</u>. Boston: Beacon Press.

Gimian, C., (2008). Beyond Carrot and Stick. <u>Shambhala Sun,</u> May, pp. 74-79.

Johnson, W. (1956). "Stuttering," pp. 216-217. In W. Johnson, *et al*. (Eds.),

    Speech Handicapped School Children, 2nd Edition. New York:

    Harper & Brothers.

Schacter-Shalomi, Z., (1997). <u>From Age-Ing to Sage-Ing</u>: <u>A Profound New</u>

    <u>Vision of Growing Older</u>. New York: Grand Central Publishing.

Seligman, M., (2004). <u>Authentic Happiness</u>. <u>Utilizing the New Positive</u>

    <u>Psychology to Realize Your Potential for Lasting Fulfillment</u>.

    New York: Free Press.

Silverman, E.-M., (2006). A Personal Choice. <u>The ASHA Leader</u>, Vol. 11 (16), p. 47.

Silverman, E.-M., (2005). *Shenpa*, Stuttering, and Me. Presented at the 8th

    Annual International Stuttering Awareness Day Online Conference, October.

Silverman, E.-M., (2003). My Personal Experience with Stuttering and

    Meditation. Presented at the 6th Annual International ISAD Online

    Conference, October.

Tolle, E., (2005). <u>A New Earth</u>. <u>Awakening to Your Life's Purpose</u>. New York:

    Penguin Group.

CD's & Videos

Chödrön, P. (2006). <u>True Happiness</u>. Boulder, Colorado: Sounds True.

Hahn, T. N. (2004). <u>The Ultimate Dimension</u>. Boulder, Colorado: Sounds True.

Kornfield, J., (2008). The Wise Heart. A Guide to the Universal Teachings of

    Buddhist Psychology (Abridged). Boulder, Colorado: Sounds True.

La Roche, L., (1995), The Joy of STRESS. Boston: WGBH/PBS.

Myss, C., (1997). Why People Don't Heal and How They Can. PBS.

END NOTES

Chapter 1

[1] *I interchange the titles therapist, clinician, and speech-language pathologist throughout. All have been and are being used, and each designates the individual who commits to providing assistance to clients and caregivers working to optimize their communication, cognitive, literacy, and/or swallowing. Some prefer therapist as a professional title because it contains within its etymology commitment to healing and cure. Others may wish to avoid such implications regarding the nature of their work and choose to identify themselves as speech-language pathologists because the profession they represent is referred to as speech-language pathology, while those engaging in a client-centered approach often preferred to be referred to as a clinician.*

[2] *I interchange the terms client and patient. Each refers to the individual involved in a process to induce maximally effective communicative, cognitive, literacy, and/or swallowing skills. The term patient is a derivative of medical practice and is often descriptive of what is expected of the recipient of medical attention, i.e., patience. The term client designates a partner in an egalitarian relationship, co-sharing responsibility with the provider of services to actively develop desired skills. Occasionally, I use the term consumer in reference to client or patient since each is a user of the service we provide and has comparable rights and responsibilities to any other consumer in the marketplace.*

Chapter 2

[1] *Rescuing (with a capital "R") occurs when an individual, i.e., the Rescuer, undertakes bold action to save another from his or her presumed plight. The antecedents require that the Rescuer believe the targeted individual incapable of surviving, let alone functioning adequately without such intervention and that the Rescuer is the one, possibly the only one, capable of such heroic service. In actuality, these are myths concocted, usually subconsciously, by Rescuers to meet their own needs, as in the vignette of the fabled boy scout who dragged an elderly woman across a busy intersection she had no intention of crossing just so he could appear helpful. It is akin to the motivation and actions of would-be martyrs. Rescuing obviates our ability to solve our own problems, thereby, negatively skews our self-concept, lessening our sense of self-sufficiency (e.g., Berne,1996).*

[2] *Partnering (with a capital "P") enjoys and encourages mutual collaboration. In clinical service, Partnering implies egalitarian functioning with each partner bringing to bear their own strengths and commitment to resolve targeted issues.*

[3] *Victim (with a capital "V")refers to a role played by someone seeking a dependency relationship in order to avoid personal responsibility and/or denigrate another by proving them incapable of successfully satisfying their needs. Again, see Berne (1966).*

[4] *Persecutor (with a capital P)is a role played by one who seeks to shame and humiliate another in order to feel good. This is an alternate role in the Rescue Game which begins with one party assuming the role of Rescuer and the other the role of Victim. During the course of the game, one of the two changes*

roles to become Persecutor, after which the game ends with both individual's covert needs seemingly met (Berne, 1996).

[5]*Please see the "Projection" section in Chapter 1.*

Chapter 3

[1]*Very few programs in speech-language pathology require or offer a course in counseling, although, increasingly programs are recommending courses in counseling taught in education or psychology departments to graduate students. Contrast this with the teaching of research design to speech-language pathology majors: Most speech-language pathology programs offer, even require, an in-house course in research design. Consequently, there are several textbooks on the subject for speech-language pathology courses, while few counseling textbooks have been published for speech-language pathologists. Altogether, these observations direct us toward the conclusion that speech-language pathologists treat by precisely and reliably counting and measuring rather than by attending to and managing feelings, their own and those of clients and caregivers (e.g., Gottfred, 2008). This is a proclivity that, like all left-brain dominated activity, soon may disappear (e.g., Pink, 2006). While bringing a sense of rationality to clinical care can help refine clients' and caregivers' perceptions of personal difficulties and treatment options, including the economics of clinical service, a so-called objective orientation to care disturbs at least as much as it encourages speech and language consumers to participate wholly in their treatment (e.g., Charon, 2006; Moore, 2006).*

Chapter 4

[1]*The term globally aphasic communicates that an individual so designated lacks the ability to encode or decode symbols and, therefore, lacks the ability to use language in all its forms, i.e., reading, writing, speaking, listening, telling time, doing arithmetic, and so forth.*

[2]*I refer to this client as Burt/Roberta because I treated both Burt and Roberta. Some sessions, few in number, I worked with Burt. Most of were spent with Roberta dressed as she felt most comfortable and true to herself.*

[3]*Lacking instruction in techniques of personal prayer until fairly recently, learning of others' pain and suffering without knowledge of the wherewithal to lessen or remove it left me feeling bereft and, generally, emotionally and physically drained as I suffered along with or for them.*

[4]*The suggestion from quantum physics that no valid distinction can be made between observer and observed suggests a drastic reorganization may be needed of our concept of "objectivity" in research and clinical work.*

Chapter 5

[1]*Organizing research efforts to satisfy statistical group research design requirements provides insights into tendencies affecting presumably isolated variables that, after they accumulate through replication,*

provide some direction for diagnosis and treatment. Field research and case studies, on the other hand, offer a broader picture of thinking and behavior of interest in milieus of interest and, therefore, more readily correspond to clinical circumstances. We need much more of this type of research to provide best practices data currently lacking.

[2]*Please read or re-read Chapter 2, "Rescuing, No. Partnering, Yes."*

[3]*Eric Berne, founder of Transactional Analysis (e.g., Berne, 1996) introduced the concept he labeled psychological game. This refers to a relationship customarily between two entities where each maintains a covert agenda designed to get them a psychological payoff they desire from the other. The game may take second, minutes, days, months, or even years to fully play-out. One such game, which is commonly played unwittingly by clinicians and clients is The Rescue Game.*

Chapter 6

[1]*That is true of clients as well. Learning how to relate skillfully to anger directed our way is useful training.*

Chapter 7

[1]*I interchange the terms patience and endurance because, in a practical sense, they are synonymous with endurance implying an expression of patience. To lessen expectations and yearnings to live fully in the present accepting what available internally and externally leads to durable change while endurance, the determination to continue exhibiting such patience, helps get us there.*

[2]*Appendix B contains an account of the development of my mindfulness, or vispassana, meditation practice documenting the fluid path such a practice can assume. The book, Coming to Our Senses by Jon Kabat-Zinn (Kabat-Zinn, 2005) well documents the various expressions of this practice.*

REFERENCES

Acredolo, L. and Goodwyn, S., (1996). <u>Baby Signs</u>. New York: Contemporary Books.

Ahlskog, G. (2001). *Reclaiming Freud's Seven Articles of Faith.* <u>Journal of Pastoral Care</u>, 55 (2).

Bennett, W. (1993). <u>The Book of Virtues</u>. New York: Simon & Schuster, Inc.

Berne, E. (1996). <u>Games People Play</u>. New York: Ballantine, Re-Issue Edition.

Berne, E. (1977). <u>Intuition and Ego States: The Origins of Transactional Analysis: A Series of Papers.</u> New York: HarperCollins.

Bloodstein, O. (1995). <u>A Handbook on Stuttering.</u> San Diego: Singular Publishing Company.

Boorstein, S. (2005). *Many Thanks.* <u>Shambhala Sun</u>, May.

Byrne, R. (2006). <u>The Secret</u>. New York: Beyond Words.

Bosnak, R. (1986). <u>A Little Course in Dreams</u>. Boston: Shambhala Publications, Inc.

Cacioppo, J. and Patrick, W. (2008). <u>Loneliness</u>. New York: W. W. Norton Company, Inc..

Campbell, J. (1988). <u>The Power of Myth</u>. New York: Broadway Books.

Carroll, M. (2007). <u>The Mindful Leader</u>. <u>Ten Principles for Bringing Out the Best In Ourselves and Others</u>. Boston: Trumpeter.

Charon, R. (2006). <u>Narrative Medicine</u>. <u>Honoring the Stories of Illness</u>. New York: Oxford Press.

Chess, S. and Thomas, A., (2005). <u>Temperament in Clinical Practice</u>. New York: The Guilford Press.

Chödrön, P. (2007). *Turn Your Thinking Upside Down.* <u>Shambhala Sun</u>, May, pp. 58-63: 105.

Chödrön, P. (2005c). <u>Practicing Peace in Times of War</u>. Boston: Shambhala Publications, Inc. (Audio CD)

Chödrön, P. (2005b). <u>Getting Unstuck</u>. Boulder, Colorado: Sounds True. (Audio CD)

Chödrön, P. (2005a). <u>No Time To Lose</u>. Boston: Shambhala Publications, Inc.

Chödrön, P. (2003). *How We Get Hooked.* <u>Shambhala Sun</u>, March.

Chödrön, P. (2000). When Things Fall Apart: Heart Advice for Difficult Times. Boston: Shambhala Publications.

Churchill, W. (1950). Painting as a Pastime. Bel Air, California: Whittlesey House.

Coffey, M. (2008). Explorers of the Infinite: The Secret Spiritual Lives of Extreme Athletes – and What They Reveal About Near-Death Experiences, Psychic Communication, and Touching the Beyond. New York: Jeremy P. Tarcher.

Crane, D. R., Griffin, W., and Hill, D. (1986). *Influence of Therapist Skills on Client Perceptions of Marriage and Family Therapy Outcome Implications For Supervision.* Journal of Marital and Family Therapy. Vol 12 (1), 91-96.

Crick, F. (1994). The Astonishing Hypothesis. The Scientific Search for the Soul New York: Charles Scribners' Sons.

Das, S. (2003). Letting Go of the Person You Used to Be. New York: Broadway Books.

Dossey, L. (2006). The Extraordinary Healing Power of Ordinary Things: Fourteen Natural Steps to Health and Happiness. New York: Harmony Books.

Dossey, L, and Myss, C. (1998). Energy Medicine. Boulder, Colorado: Sounds True.

Dyer, W. (2007). Change Your Thinking. Change Your Life: Living the Wisdom of the Tao. Carlsbad, California: Hay House.

Edwards, B. (2001). The New Drawing on the Right Side of the Brain, 3rd Edition. New York: Harper Collins Publishers, Ltd.

Eisenson, J. (Ed.) (1958). STUTTERING: A Symposium. New York: Harper & Row Publisher.

Emoto, M. (2004). The Hidden Messages in Water. Hillsboro, Oregon: Beyond Words Publishing, Inc.

Fehmi, L, and Robbins, J. (2007). The Open Focus Brain: Harnessing the Power of Attention to Heal Mind and Body. Boston: Trumpeter.

Fontana, D. (1999). Learn to Meditate. San Francisco: Chronicle Books.

Fontana, D., and Slack, I. (1998). Teaching Meditation to Children: A Practical Guide to the Use and Benefits of Meditation Techniques. New York: Element Books.

Frankl, V., (2006). Man's Search for Meaning. Boston: Beacon Press.

Friedman, R. (2007). *Understanding Empathy: Can You Feel My Pain?* New York Times, *Health*, April 24, p. 5.

Gafni, M. (2004). <u>The Soul Prints Workshop: Wisdom Teachings from the Kabbalah Illuminating Your Unique Life Purpose</u>. Boulder, Colorado: Sounds True. (Audio CD)

Gimian, C., (2008). *Beyond Carrot and Stick*. <u>Shambhala Sun,</u> May, pp. 74-79.

Gladwell, M., (2007). <u>Blink</u>. New York: Back Bay Books.

Goleman, D. (2006a). *I Feel Your Brain*. <u>Tricycle</u>. Winter, pp. 66-69; 118-119.

Goleman, D. (2006b). <u>Social Intelligence</u>. <u>The New Science of Human Relationships</u>. New York: Bantam.

Gottfred, K., (2008). *Scientifically Based Professional Practice*. <u>The ASHA Leader</u>, 13 (16), pp. 26-27.

Groopman, J. (2007). <u>How Doctors Think</u>. New York: Houghton Mifflin Company.

Grossman, L. (2007). *"Bill Gates Goes Back to School."* <u>Time</u>, Vol. 162 (25), pp. 46-48.

Hanh, T. (2004). <u>The Ultimate Dimension</u>. Boulder, Colorado: Sounds True. (Audio CD)

Hanh, T. N. (2000). <u>The Wisdom of Thich Nhat Hanh</u>. <u>The Sun in My Heart</u>, pp. 335-334. Mechanicsburg, Pennsylvania: Book-of-the-Month Club, Inc.

Hanh, T. N. (1992). <u>Peace is Every Step</u>. New York: Bantam.

Harris, T., (2004). <u>I'm OK. You're OK</u>. New York: Harper Paperbacks.

H.H. the Dalai Lama, (2006). <u>How to See YOURSELF As You Really Are</u>. New York: Atria Books.

H.H. the Dalai Lama, (2005a). <u>How to Expand Love</u>. *Widening the Circle of Loving* <u>Relationships</u>. New York: Atria Books.

H.H. the Dalai Lama (2005b). <u>The Universe in a Single Atom</u>. <u>The Convergence Of Science and Spirituality</u>. New York: Morgan Books.

Hellman, L., (2000). *<u>Pentimento</u>*. New York: Back Bay Books. (Reissue Edition)

Heschel, A. (2005). <u>The Sabbath</u>. New York: Farrar, Strauss, Giroux.

Hinckley, J. (2007). <u>Narrative-Based Practice in Speech-Language Pathology</u>: <u>Stories of a Clinical Life</u>. San Diego, CA.: Plural Publishing.

Jung, C. (1997). <u>Man and His Symbols</u>. New York: Dell.

Jung, C. (1976). <u>The Portable Jung</u>. New York: Penguin.

Kabat-Zinn, J. (2006). Mindfulness for Beginners. Boulder, Colorado: Sounds True.

Kabat-Zinn, J. (2005). Coming to Our Senses. Healing Ourselves and The World Through Mindfulness. New York: Hyperion.

Kabat-Zinn, J. (1995). Wherever You Go, There You Are: Mindfulness Meditation in Everyday Life. New York Hyperion.

Katie, B. (2007). Your Inner Awakening. The Work of Byron Katie. Four Questions That Will Transform Your Life (Unabridged). Niles, Illinois: Nightingale-Conant. (Audio CD)

Katie, B. (2003). Loving What Is: Four Questions that Can Change Your Life. New York: Three Rivers Press.

Kelly, W. (1987). Pogo: We Have Met the Enemy and He is Us. New York: Simon & Schuster.

Kisilevsky, B., Hains, S., Kang, L., Xie, X., Huang, H., Ye, H., Zhuang, K., and Wang, Z., (2003). Effects of Experience on Fetal Voice Recognition. Psychological Science. Vol. 14 (3), 220-224.

Kliewer, S. (2004). Allowing Spirituality into the Healing Process. Journal of Family Practice,, 53, 616-624.

Kongtrul, D. (2006). It's Up to You. Boston: Shambhala Publications.

Kornfield, J. (2003). The Inner Art of Meditation. Boulder, Colorado: Sounds True.

Kornfield, J. (2005). Meditation for Beginners. Boulder, Colorado: Sounds True.

Korzybski, A. (1955). Science and Sanity, 5th Edition. Fort Worth, Texas: Institute of General Semantics.

Kubler-Ross, E. (1997). On Death and Dying. New York: Scribner.

Kushner, H. (2006). Overcoming Life's Disappointments. New York: Alfred A. Knopf.

Lad, V. (1994). AyurVeda. Boulder, Colorado: Sounds True.

La Roche, L. (2002). The Joy of Stress with Loretta La Roche. Boston: WGBH. (VHS Tape)

Langer, E. (1989). Mindfulness. Reading, Massachusetts: Addison-Wesley Publishing Company, Inc.

Liebovich, M. (2007). Listening and Nodding, Clinton Shapes '08 Image. New York Times, March 6, p.1; p.18.

Lipton, B. (2005). The Biology of Belief. Unleashing the Power of Consciousness, Matter, and Miracles. Santa Rosa, California: Mountain of Love.

Lorenz, K., and Kickert, R. (2004). The Foundations of Ethology. New York: Springer Publishing Company.

Malchiodi, C. (Ed.) (2002). Handbook of Art Therapy. New York: Guilford Press.

Maroda, K. (1991). The Power of Countertransference. Innovations in Analytic Technique. New York: John Wiley & Sons.

Mipham, S. (2007). *There is no 'I' in happy.* Shambhala Sun, March, 19-20.

Mipham, S. (2006). Ruling Your World. Ancient Strategies for Modern Life. New York: Morgan Road Books.

Moore, L. (2006). *Empathy: A Clinician's Perspective.* The ASHA Leader, 11(10), 16-17; 34-35.

Mother Teresa and Kolodiejchuk, B. (2007). Mother Teresa: Come Be My Light. New York: Doubelday.

Mueller, W. (1999). Sabbath: Finding Rest, Renewal, and Delight in Our Busy Lives. New York: Bantam.

Myers, I. with P. Myers (1995). Gifts Differing: Understanding Personality Type. Mountain View, CA: Davies-Black Publishing.

Myss, C. (2004b). Why People Don't Heal and How They Can/Three Levels of Power and How to se Them. Wellspring Media.

Myss, C., (2004a). Essential Guide for Healers. Boulder, Colorado: Sounds True. (Audio CD)

Myss, C., (2002c). Spiritual Madness. Boulder, Colorado: Sounds True. (Audio CD)

Myss, C., (2002b). Self-Esteem. Your Fundamental Power. Boulder, Colorado: Sounds True. (Audio CD)

Myss, C. (2002a). Sacred Contracts. New York: Harmony Books.

Myss, C. (1997). Anatomy of the Spirit: The Seven Stages of Power and Healing. New York: Three Rivers Press.

Nguyen, A. H. and Hanh, T. N. (2006). Walking Meditation. Boulder, Colorado: Sounds True. (Includes a CD and a DVD)

Orloff, J. (2004). Positive Energy. New York: Harmony Books.

Ornstein, R. (1996). The Mind Field: A Personal Essay. Reprint Edition. Boston: Malor Books.

Pedulla, T. (2008). *Jets Confidence Building Keyed by Favre's Composure.* USA Today Online, (November 28).

Pink, D. (2006). A Whole New Mind: Why Right-Brainers Will Rule the Future, *Up-Dated Edition*. New York: Riverhead Trade Books.

Pitchford, P. (2002). Healing With Whole Foods, 3rd Edition. Berkeley, California: North Atlantic Books.

Progoff, I. (1983). Life Study: Experiencing Creative Lives by the Intensive Journal Method. New York: Dialogue House Library.

Progroff, I. (1975). At A Journal Workshop. New York: Jeremy Tarcher.

Quesal, R., (2001). *The Death of Fluency Disorders.* Presented at the 4th International ISAD Online Conference, October. (Accessible at http://www.mnsu.edu/comdis/kuster/stutter.html)

Ray, R. (2003). Meditating with the Body. Boulder, Colorado: Sounds True. (Audio CD)

Richo, D. (2008). When the Past is Present: Healing Emotional Wounds that Sabotage Our Relationships. Boston: Shambhala Publications.

Rogers, C. (1996). On Becoming A Person: A Therapist's View of Psychotherapy. Gloucester, MA: Peter Smith Publisher.

Rosenberg, M. (2004). Raising Children Compassionately: Parenting the Nonviolent Communication Way. Encinitas, California: Puddledancer Press.

Rosenberg, M. (2003). Nonviolent Communication: A Language of Life: Create Your Life, Your Relationships, and Your World in Harmony with Your Values. Encinitas, California: Puddledancer Press.

Rozman, D. (2002). Meditating With Children – The Art of Concentration and Centering: A Workbook on New Educational Methods Using Meditation. Virginia: Integral Yoga Publications.

Salzberg, S., and Goldstein, J. (2002). Insight Meditation: A Step-by-Step Course On How To Meditate. Boulder, Colorado: Sounds True. (Audio CD)

Sarton, M. (2002). Journal of A Solitude. New York: W.W. Norton & Company.

Schulz, M., and Northrup, C. (2005). <u>The New Feminine Brain: How Women Can Develop Their Inner Strengths, Genius, and Intuition</u>. New York: Free Press.

Shafir, R. (2000). <u>The Zen of Listening: Mindful Communication in the Age of Distraction</u>. Wheaton, Illinois: Theosophical Publishing House.

Shealy, C.N. and Myss, C. (1988). <u>Creation of Health: Merging Traditional Medicine with Intuitive Diagnosis</u>. Walpole, New Hampshire: Stillpoint Publishing.

Sheldrake, R. (1982). <u>A New Science of Life.</u> New York: J. P. Tarcher.

Siegel, B. (1986). <u>Love, Medicine, & Miracles</u>. New York: Harper & Row.

Siegel, S. and E. Lowe, Jr. (1992). <u>The Patient Who Cured His Therapist.</u> <u>And Other Tales of Therapy</u>. New York: Dutton.

Silverman, E.-M. (2009). *Doing the Work*. Paper presented at the 12th Annual ISAD International Online Conference, October.

Silverman, E.-M. (2008c). *Happily Ever After*. Paper presented at the 11th Annual ISAD International Online Conference, October. (See Appendix C).

Silverman, E.-M. (2008b). *Ongoing Self-Reflection*. <u>American Journal of Speech-Language Pathology</u>, 17 (1), 92.

Silverman, E.-M. (2008a). *Applying Narrative Techniques*. *The ASHA Leader*, Vol. 13 (2), 46.

Silverman, E.-M. (2007b). *The Pain Issue.* <u>Shambhala Sun</u>, July, p. 17.

Silverman, E.-M. (2007a). Creating Conditions for Change. Paper presented at the 10th Annual ISAD International Online Conference, October. (Accessible at <u>http://www.mnsu.edu/comdis/kuster/stutter.html</u> and included in its entirety in Appendix A.)

Silverman, E.-M. (2006c). *Mind Matters*. Paper presented at the 9th Annual ISAD International Online Conference, October. (Accessible at <u>http://www.mnsu.edu/comdis/kuster/stutter.html</u>)

Silverman, E.-M. (2006b). *Empathy and Compassion*. <u>The ASHA Leader</u>, 11(16), 4.

Silverman, E. -M. (2006a). *A Personal Choice*. <u>The ASHA Leader</u>. 11(15), 47.

Silverman, E.-M. (2005)*, Shenpa, Stuttering, and Me*. 8th Annual International ISAD Online Conference, October. (Accessible at <u>http://www.mnsu.edu/comdis/kuster/stutter.html</u>)

Silverman, E.-M (2004). *Using Story to Help Heal*. Paper Presented a the 7th Annual International ISAD Online Conference. October. (Accessible at http://www.mnsu.edu/comdis/kuster/stutter.html)

Silverman, E.-M. (2003d). *My Personal Experience with Stuttering and Meditation*. 6th Annual International ISAD Online Conference, October. (Accessible at http://www.mnsu.edu/comdis/kuster/stutter.html)

Silverman, E.-M. (2003c). *A Clinical Profession?* The ASHA Leader. 8 (1), 23.

Silverman, E.-M. (2003b). *Where We Are Going?* The ASHA Leader. 8, (4), 29.

Silverman, E. -M. (2003a). *Shared Connections - Spirituality in Clinical Practice*. The ASHA Leader. *Guest Editorial*. 8 (17), 40.

Silverman, E.-M. (2001c). *Consumer Alert*: Stuttering and Gender Research 4th Annual International ISAD Online Conference, October. (Accessible at http://www.mnsu.edu/comdis/kuster/stutter.html)

Silverman, E.-M. (2001b). *Clinical Preparation and Clinical Effectiveness*. The ASHA Leader, 6, p. 23.

Silverman, E.-M. (2001a). Jason's Secret. Indianapolis: 1st Books.

Silverman, E.-M. (2000). *Our Image*. American Journal of Speech-Language Pathology, Vol. 9, 172-173.

Silverman, E.-M. (1992). *Integrating Counseling Skills into Speech-Language Pathology And Audiology*. A Miniseminar Presented at The Annual Meeting of the American Speech-Language-Hearing Association, San Antonio.

Silverman, E.-M. (1979). *You and I*. Unpublished poem.

Silverman, E.-M. (1970). *A Study of The Disfluency Behavior of 10 Four-Year-Old Males*. *Doctoral Dissertation*. The University of Iowa.

Simon, T., (Ed.) (2008). Measuring the Immeasurable: The Scientific Case for Spirituality. Boulder, Colorado: Sounds True, Inc.

Sohan, T. (2008). *Redefining Leadership*. The ASHA Leader, Vol 13 (30), p. 39.

Soygal, R. (2005). Tibetan Wisdom for Living and Dying. Boulder, Colorado: ounds True. (Audio CD)

Spillers, C. (2007). *An Existential Framework for Understanding the Counseling Needs of Clients*. American Journal of Speech-Language Pathology. Vol. 16 (3), 191-197.

Stein, J., (2003). *Just Say Om*. Time Magazine, August 4.

Steiner, C. (1990). Scripts People Live. Grove/Atlantic. Reprint Edition.

Steinsaltz, A. (2002). A Guide to Jewish Prayer. New York: Schocken Books.

Storr, A. (1989). Solitude: A Return to the Self. New York: Ballentine Books.

Tannen, D. (2001). You Just Don't Understand: Women and Men in Conversation. New York: Harper Paperbacks.

Telushkin, J. (1998). Words that Hurt, Words that Heal: How to Choose Words Wisely and Well. New York: Harper Paperbacks.

Tsu, L. (1989). Tao Te Ching. New York: Vintage Publishing.

Tuma, R. (2007). *What Monks Know and We Can Learn About the Fruits of Meditation*. Yoga Plus, May-June, pp. 38-42.

Van Riper, C. (1973). The Treatment of Stuttering. Englewood Cliffs, N.J.: Prentice-Hall.

Wangyal, T. (2006). Tibetan Sound Healing. Boulder: Boulder, Colorado: Sounds True.(Audio CD)

Weil, A. (1995). Spontaneous Healing. New York: Alfred A. Kopf.

Wiegela, K. (1996). How to Be a Help Rather Than a Nuisance: Practical Approaches to Giving Support, Service, and Encouragement to Others. Boston: Shambhala

Williams, M. (2003). Learning Their Language. Novato, California: New World Library.

Wiseman, R. (2003). Queen Bees and Wannabes: Helping Your Daughter Survive, Cliques, Gossip, Boyfriends, and Other Realities of Adolescence. New York: Three Rivers Press.

Woodruff, L., and Woodruff, B. (2007). In an Instant: A Family's Journey of Love And Healing. New York: Random House.

Zukav, G., (1999). The Seat of the Soul. New York: Simon and Schuster.

ABOUT THE AUTHOR

Ellen-Marie Silverman began her career in 1964 as a speech correctionist in an experimental program for autistic preschoolers. Realizing she had much to learn, she entered the University of Iowa 15 months later as a graduate student in Speech Pathology. By the summer of 1969, she had earned both an M.A. and a Ph.D. from that university. Still not feeling fully prepared for clinical work, she undertook a post-doctoral fellowship in developmental psycholinguistics at the University of Illinois, Urbana-Champaign, then joined the University's Institute of Communications Research as a research associate. That began her career in academia which spanned 15 years and included membership on the Marquette University and The Medical College of Wisconsin faculties. Dr. Silverman has published extensively in professional journals and has presented at local, state, national, and international meetings. She is a Fellow of the American Speech-Hearing-Language Association.

Returning to full-time clinical service in 1985, she has, during the course of her clinical career, provided service to inpatient and outpatient rehabilitation settings, a private day school, skilled nursing facilities, and home health in addition to maintaining a private practice. Having been a Transactional Analysis trainee from 1980 to 1981 and 1984-1985, she utilized what she learned about personality and fashioning useful clinical relationships to revitalize her work. She eventually founded and operated TSS-The Speech Source, Inc., a multi-faceted staffing service that provided temporary occupational, physical, and speech therapy services as well as interpreting and captioning, including live theater captioning, which she pioneered in Wisconsin.

Dr. Silverman authored *Jason's Secret*, a novel about stuttering for children aged 9-12. Readers learn Jason's thoughts and feelings as a fifth grader in a new school learning to face, rather than conceal, his stuttering problem, speak with greater ease and skill, and express anger constructively. She wrote the book to help release children with stuttering problems from a not uncommon sense of isolation, demystify speech therapy, and help interested and caring adults, siblings, and classmates better understand what it feels like to have a stuttering problem and what it can take to overcome one.

INDEX

A

Acredolo 137

Ahlskog 63, 77

Allione 45, 185, 186

Altman 61, 62

American Speech-Language-Hearing Association 79

Anger 25, 28 ,29, 43, 44, ,46, 57, 67, 71, 102, 103, 104, 107, 108, 117, 131, 132, 138, 145, 149, 183, 191

Appearance 66, 77, 89, 90, 114

Archetypes 34, 49

ASHA 54, 141

Asking and Answering Why? 26, 27, 30, 77, 157, 158, 159

Attending 32, 73, 86, 87, 88, 95, 99, 150, 156, 160, 190

Autism 16, 17

Avoidance 118, 185

B

Behaviorist 95

Being Present 32, 88, 154

Being Right 31, 125, 126

Berne 63, 96, 103, 104, 118, 125

Bloodstein 133

Bon Buddhist Tradition 33

Bontrager 26

Boorstein 170

Bosnak 34, 98

Brain Injury 13, 14, 17, 18, 19, 24, 64, 65, 66, 74, 86, 101, 102, 120, 121-122, 136

Buddha 39, 42, 79, 97, 107

Burn-Out 2, 12, 71

Byrne 77, 171

C

Cabbalists 101

Cacioppo 171

Carroll 153

Certainties 21, 22, 24, 26, 34, 132

Change 3, 4, 6, 25, 27, 29, 29, 30, 31, 33, 34, 36, 37, 38, 39, 40, 41, 42, 43, 44, 46

Charon 23, 34, 55, 135, 138, 190

Chassidic Rabbis 40

Chess 137, 168, 169, 171

Chödrön 20, 33, 43, 77, 92, 93, 103, 113, 132, 154, 157, 179, 185

Churchill 161

Clinical Decision-Making 2, 73, 89, 92

Clinical Fellowship Year 72, 135, 139

Clinical Role 49, 51

Clinician 1, 3, 4, 5, 9, 22, 25, 51, 52, 89, 120, 123, 125, 139, 146, 161, 184, 189, 191

Clinton 87, 88

Code of Ethics 1

Coffey 96

Collaborators 53, 123

Collective Unconscious 34

Community 33, 40, 41, 87, 93, 97, 105, 126, 146, 170, 185

Compassion 2, 6, 12, 16, 40, 41, 42, 43, 45, 46, 47, 81, 86, 105, 118, 119, 137

Conditioned Thinking 90

Consumer 122, 189, 190

Contracting 31, 67, 69

Core Beliefs 1, 3, 4, 5, 9, 12, 20, 21, 22, 24, 25, 26, 31, 34, 38, 76, 92, 110, 139, 154, 157

Counseling 24, 79, 102, 125, 139, 140, 141, 190

Counter-transference 15, 16

Crane 23

D

Dakini Bliss 43

Dalai Lama 23, 77, 92, 101

Das 38
Dean Williams 89
Dharma 178
Dossey 96
DuBois 84
Dyer 125
Dysphagia 133
Dysphonia 30

E
Edwards 160
Einstein 22, 83, 115, 122, 151
Emerson 171
Emoto 24
Empathy 11, 12, 19, 86, 98, 99, 100, 106
Empathetic 2, 11, 47, 53, 60, 86, 96, 98, 99, 100, 101, 102, 103
Endurance 3, 6, 39, 79, 143, 146, 147, 148, 151, 152, 153, 155, 157, 159, 161, 171, 191
Energy Vampires 103
Epigenetics 22
Evidence Based Practice 75
Expectation 13, 14, 20, 43, 54, 64, 67, 68, 72, 88, 100, 105, 122, 125, 155, 179, 184, 191

F
Fable 131
Fix 51, 52, 53, 67, 148
Follow-Through 91, 145
Fontana 33, 156
Freud 63, 101, 126

G
Gafni 20, 163
Gandhi 20
General Semantics 26, 129, 160
Gimian 46, 186
Gladwell 23
Golden Rule 105, 106

Goldstein 33, 92
Goleman 20, 23, 24, 71, 99, 105
Gottsfred 75
Gratitude 34, 111, 158, 159, 177
Gratitude Journal 111
Groopman 89
Grossman 127
Guard-All 99, 102, 103, 104

H
Habitual Behavior 78
Hanh 32, 93, 132, 150, 153, 184, 185
Happiness 3, 45, 72, 76, 94, 114, 137, 140, 181, 183, 185, 186
Harris 45
Hasidic Jews 46, 114
Havdalah 152
Heal 84
Healing 25, 33, 68, 86, 87, 99, 100, 119, 159, 185
Hellman 110, 123, 170, 171
Heschel 152
Hinckley 1
Hopkins 21
Huston 80

I
Imprinting 138
Indulgence 45, 46
Insight Meditation 33, 92
International Online Conference 27
Intuition 29, 30, 95, 96
Intuitive Reception 98
ISAD 7, 27, 80, 94, 165

J
Jewish Geography 83, 84
Journaling 5, 26, 31, 34, 42, 152, 156, 157, 158, 159
Jones 76, 77
Joyce 31
Jung 23, 34, 79, 96, 126

K

Kabat-Zinn 5, 32, 33, 92, 110, 140, 153, 156
Kabbalah 87
Kabbalists 163
Katie 92, 93, 110, 150
Kelly 136
Kickert 138
Kindness 11, 12, 15, 41, 42, 43, 45, 51, 81, 84, 94, 99, 106, 119, 148, 157, 186
Kisilevsky 138
Kolodiejchuk 146
Kongtrül 42, 43
Kornfield 4, 33, 87, 92, 93, 103, 153, 184
Korzybski 26, 115, 160
Kubler-Ross 96
Kushner 22
Kuster 3, 7, 167, 183

L

Lao Tsu 125
La Roche 33, 185
Langer 20, 32
Leibovich 88
Lipton 20, 22, 97, 101
Listening 11, 45, 50, 61, 69, 78, 86, 87, 88, 112, 150, 153, 154
Litigation 20, 29, 67, 85, 135
Lorenz 138

M

Malchiodi 162
Maroda 14, 16
Martyr 49, 189
MBSR 33, 92, 140
Meditation 20, 26, 32, 33, 42, 43, 44, 55, 77, 92, 96, 97, 103, 132, 152, 153, 154, 155, 156, 159, 175, 177
Meditating 43, 93, 152, 153, 154, 155, 159, 160, 177, 179
McGraw 84, 125

Milarepa 44, 45
Mind 59, 80, 86, 92, 93, 94, 98, 99, 101, 105, 107, 123, 132, 146, 151, 152, 153, 154, 159, 160, 163, 165, 170, 171
Mindfully 143
Mindfulness 26, 31, 32, 33, 34, 92, 96, 98, 103, 140, 153, 154, 159, 175, 179, 191
Mindfulness Based Stress Reduction 33, 92, 140
Mindfulness Practice 154
Mipham 76, 92, 93, 112, 151, 152
Moore 98, 190
Mother Theresa 146, 148
Motives 14, 65, 86, 110, 156
Muller 152
Myer-Briggs 96
Myers 96
Myss 34, 37, 41, 98, 102, 104, 110, 116, 170, 171
Mystics 101

N

Narrative Medicine 34
Nin 88, 101
Northrup 71, 96, 98
Nyguyen 155

O

Objective 23, 95, 110, 128, 129, 190
Objectivity 129, 190
O.K. 76, 78, 79
Organizing Beliefs 1
Orloff 96, 98, 103, 112

P

Painting 22, 110, 152, 153, 155, 159, 160, 161, 162
Partner 18, 21, 32, 38, 49, 50, 51, 53, 58, 60, 61, 62, 68, 69, 79, 87, 88, 93, 100, 104, 122, 123, 126, 138, 148, 170
Partnering 15, 47, 49, 51, 52, 53, 61, 62, 63, 67, 69, 85, 91, 126, 138, 139, 148

Patience 35, 36, 94, 99, 113, 143, 145, 146, 147, 148, 149, 152, 158, 161, 167, 177

Patrick 178

Prayer 42, 44, 57, 111, 152, 190

Pedulla 80

Pema Chödrön 20, 43, 132, 154, 179, 185

Perls 13

Permission 63, 65

Persecutor 60, 61

Placebos 22

Placebo Effect 22

Pink 75, 190

Pity 19, 46, 53, 85, 100, 114

Playing Politics 73, 74

Potency 63

Professional Burn-Out 12

Projection 12, 46, 50, 71, 101, 154, 190

Protection 63, 65, 71

Progroff 34, 159

Proxemics 138

Q

Quantum Mechanics 101, 129, 149

Quantum Theory 101

R

Ray 43, 79, 88, 93

Reflection 28, 41, 42, 74, 92, 94, 99, 101, 113, 156

Relationships 15, 16, 21, 28, 58, 72, 73, 74, 75, 87, 110, 122, 125, 136, 137, 140, 145, 170, 171, 178

Rescue Game 123

Rescuer 30, 49, 50, 51, 53, 57, 58, 60, 61, 63, 65, 68, 96, 148

Resistance 136, 140, 185

Rescuing 47, 49, 50, 51, 52, 53, 54, 148

Richo 13, 14

Right View 130

Rose 76, 153, 161

Rozman 156

Rosenberg 132, 137

S

Sabbath 152

Safety 24, 41, 65, 91, 104

Salzberg 33, 92

Samurai 134

Sanders 125

Samuels 87

Sarton 31, 156

Schacter-Shalomi 183

Schultz 96, 98

Self-Acceptance 29, 77, 79, 80

Self-Awareness 33, 50, 61, 77, 93, 162

Self-Esteem 62, 104, 118, 121, 185

Self-Knowledge 26, 29, 81, 92, 102, 156, 158

Self-Reflection 5, 9, 12, 28, 41, 42, 92, 94, 99, 113

Self-Talk 5, 21, 36, 39, 147, 150, 154, 175, 186

Self-Worth 53, 73, 74, 75, 76, 106, 122, 170

Seligman 184, 185

Shakyamuni Buddha 39, 79

Shafir 86, 154

Shealy 96

Sheldrake 23

Shenpa 27, 33, 92, 103, 154, 157, 158, 175, 179

Siegel 22, 96

Silverman 11, 12, 17, 27, 32, 33, 34, 37, 41, 43, 44, 46, 58, 60, 61, 68, 77, 85, 86, 92, 93, 96, 98, 103, 106, 110, 113, 114, 118, 120, 126, 132, 134, 135, 138, 140, 141, 147, 154, 156, 157, 158, 162, 165, 169, 171

Simon 83

Sitting 19, 27, 31, 33, 65, 66, 100, 110, 122, 129, 153, 155, 177, 178, 179

Six Degrees of Kevin Bacon 83
Slack 122, 156
Sohan 2
Soygal 4
Spielberg 61, 62
Spillers 83
Spiritual 20, 54, 103, 114, 133, 134, 146, 186
Spirituality 133
Stein 93, 161
Steiner 21, 168, 169, 171
Stereotyping 15
Story 44, 87, 131, 163
Stuart 87, 88
Stuttering 13, 14, 25, 27, 28, 33, 36, 38, 39, 51, 55, 56, 57, 58, 59, 60, 73, 79, 80, 94, 118, 119, 120, 121, 123, 127, 133, 134, 146, 147, 156, 165, 167, 170, 175, 179, 181, 183, 184, 185, 186
Subconscious 14, 15, 34, 101, 159
Suffering 17, 22, 26, 85, 86, 96, 98, 99, 105, 106, 114, 124, 190
Suicide 55, 56, 57
Sufis 101
Suzuki Roshi 76
Sympathy 19, 46, 85, 86, 99, 100, 103

T
T'sen T'sang 125
TA 24, 25, 26, 47, 49, 78, 139
Tangka 153
Tannen 62
Telushkin 24
Tennessee Williams 84
The Buddha 39, 42, 97, 107, 131
Therapist 11, 12, 13, 14, 15, 16, 17, 18, 19, 24, 25, 28, 29, 33, 50, 51, 52, 54, 56, 58, 60, 61, 62, 63, 64, 65, 66, 74, 78, 79, 81, 85, 86, 90, 91, 92, 100, 116, 123, 147, 185
Theravada 97

Theravadan 178
The *Tao 105*
Thomas 6, 76, 114, 137, 168, 169, 171
Tolle 184
Tonglen 33
Torah 87, 163, 178
Transactional Analysis 21, 24, 25, 26, 31, 39, 45, 49, 63, 76, 78, 93, 96, 102, 139, 178
Transference 13, 14, 15, 16
Traumatic Brain Injury 13, 14, 17, 18, 24, 64, 65, 66, 74, 86, 101, 102, 120, 121, 122, 136
Tuma 92, 93
Tzadik 46

U
Unconscious 13, 14, 26, 34, 90, 126
Us-ness 99, 100

V
Vajrayana 178
Validation 72, 73, 88
Victim 56, 57, 58, 60, 61, 126
Vignette 36, 103, 104
Vin Diesel 168, 169, 185
Vipassana 53

W
Wangyal 201
Weil 39
Wiegela 152
Wilde 83
Williams 84, 89, 98
Winfrey 50, 71
Wiseman 75, 77
Woodruff 96, 97

Z
Zen 76, 77, 125, 150
Zukav 61, 69

www.ingramcontent.com/pod-product-compliance
Lightning Source LLC
Chambersburg PA
CBHW080229200526

45165CB00026B/3331